Paediatric
Life Support

W

Paediatric Advanced Life Support
A Practical Guide for Nurses

Second Edition

Phil Jevon RN BSc (Hons) PGCE

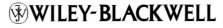
WILEY-BLACKWELL

A John Wiley & Sons, Ltd., Publication

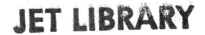

Library of Congress Cataloging-in-Publication Data

Data available

ISBN 978-14051-9776-2

A catalogue record for this book is available from the British Library.

Wiley also publishes its books in a variety of electronic formats. Some content that appears in print may not be available in electronic books.

Set in 10/12 pt Palatino by Toppan Best-set Premedia Limited
Printed and bound in Singapore by Markono Print Media Pte Ltd

[1   2012]

Contents

Foreword

The death of any child is a tragedy, but is more so if that death could have been prevented.

In England and Wales, the mortality rate for infants and children has fallen by more than 50% in the last three decades and is now at its' lowest ever level.

This fall is due in part to an increasing understanding of the causes of death in infants and children and the recognition that many of these deaths are preventable and are preceded by a recognisable period of deterioration in respiratory and circulatory function secondary to an underlying condition which is often potentially treatable. Failure to intervene early in such infants and children can lead to cardiac arrest which has a dismal outcome. This is seen most markedly by contrasting the survival rates of patients in asystole (survival rates of less than 5% being reported), with those of children in respiratory arrest who have received prompt resuscitation (survival rates of over 50% being reported).

Paediatric Advanced Life Support (PALS) is a succinct yet comprehensive guide to the knowledge, skills, drugs and equipment necessary to identify and effectively treat infants and children who have potential life threatening conditions, and thus prevent a cardiac arrest. It provides an evidence-based approach to paediatric advanced life support based on the latest Resuscitation Council UK 2010 guidelines. The text is complimented by the inclusion of the latest Resuscitation Council algorithms. The book emphasises the logical and systematic team approach required to recognise and manage the seriously ill child and provides a concise source of essential information.

This second edition is pocket sized and presents the most recent information in an accessible format and serves as an excellent reference source for all involved or potentially involved in the treatment and management of the sick child particularly nurses, junior doctors and allied health professionals. I can highly recommend it.

Derek Burke
Consultant in Paediatric Emergency Medicine
Sheffield Children's NHS Foundation Trust
UK

Contributors

Consulting Editors

Kathleen Berry, Consultant Paediatrician A & E, Birmingham Children's Hospital, Birmingham, UK

Gale Pearson, Consultant Paediatrician PICU, Birmingham Children's Hospital, Birmingham, UK

Contributors

Jayne Breakwell, Senior Sister Paediatrics, Walsall Healthcare NHS Trust, Manor Hospital, Walsall, UK

Kirsti Soanes, Matron Paediatrics, Birmingham Children's Hospital, Birmingham, UK

Richard Griffin, Lecturer in Law, Swansea University, Wales

Chapter 1

An Overview of Paediatric Advanced Life Support

Introduction

Paediatric advanced life support (PALS) includes the knowledge and skills necessary to identify and effectively treat infants and children who have potential respiratory or circulatory failure, and to provide the appropriate early treatment for a paediatric cardiac arrest.

The aim of this chapter is to provide an overview of PALS.

Learning objectives

At the end of this chapter, the reader will be able to:

- Discuss the causes of death in childhood
- Discuss survival rates following paediatric resuscitation
- Outline the pathophysiology of paediatric cardiac arrest
- Discuss the importance of treating children differently from adults
- Outline the provision of a resuscitation service in hospital

Causes of death in childhood

The most common causes of death in children under 6 years of age worldwide are detailed in Table 1.1.

Paediatric Advanced Life Support: A Practical Guide for Nurses, Second Edition.
Phil Jevon.
© 2012 Phil Jevon. Published 2012 by Blackwell Publishing Ltd.

Table 1.1 Most common causes of death worldwide in children under 6 years of age

Neonates aged 0–27 days		Children aged 1–59 months	
Preterm birth complications	12%	Diarrhoea	14%
Birth asphyxia	9%	Pneumonia	14%
Sepsis	6%	Other infections	9%
Other	5%	Malaria	8%
Pneumonia	4%	Other non-communicable disease	4%
Congenital abnormalities	3%	Injury	3%
Diarrhoea	1%	AIDS	2%
Tetanus	1%	Pertussis	2%

Reproduced from Stevenson & Tedrow (2010).

Table 1.2 Causes of death by age in England and Wales, 2008

	0–4 weeks	1–12 months	1–4 years	5–14 years
Number of deaths	3918	1023	506	590
Perinatal conditions and prematurity	62%	22%	3%	1%
Congenital	25%	20%	15%	7%
Sudden unexplained deaths	1%	19%	3%	1%
Respiratory infections	Included in 'Other infections'	6%	11%	8%
Other infections	1%	7%	11%	3%
Trauma including asphyxia	10%	4%	13%	19%
Other	1%	6%	2%	1%

Reproduced from Office for National Statistics (2010).

According to the Office for National Statistics (2009), the highest death rates in childhood occur during the first year of life, particularly the first month (Table 1.2). Causes of death in childhood vary according to age. The most common causes are:

- *Newborn period* – congenital abnormalities and factors associated with prematurity
- *1 month to 1 year* – cot death, infection and congenital abnormality
- *From 1 year* – trauma

In England and Wales, infant mortality rates (number of deaths of children under 1 year of age in one calendar year per 1000 live births in the same calendar year) have fallen by more than 50% in the last 28 years, from 12 in 1980 down to 4.5 in 2008, the lowest on record (Advanced Life Support Group, 2011).

Survival rates following paediatric resuscitation

Paediatric cardiac arrest is rarely caused by a primary cardiac problem. It is also rarely a sudden event (Klitzener, 1995), often being the end result of a progressive deterioration in respiratory and circulatory function (American Academy of Paediatrics, 2000). If cardiac arrest ensues, the prognosis is dismal (O'Rourke, 1986); the survival rate of patients in asystole has been reported to be as low as 3% (Zaritsky *et al.*, 1987).

The early diagnosis and aggressive management of respiratory or cardiac insufficiency aimed at preventing deterioration to cardiac arrest are the key to improving survival without neurological deficit in seriously ill children (Zideman & Spearpoint, 1999). Prompt resuscitation in the event of a respiratory arrest is associated with a favourable outcome – survival rates of over 50% have been reported (Zaritsky *et al.*, 1987; Spearpoint, 2002). Recognition of respiratory failure and shock is discussed in Chapter 3.

Pathophysiology of cardiac arrest

There are three basic mechanisms of paediatric cardiac arrest – asystole, pulseless electrical activity (PEA; formerly known as electromechanical dissociation) and ventricular fibrillation (VF). Pulseless ventricular tachycardia (VT) is another mechanism, but this is usually classified with VF because the causes and treatment are similar.

Asystole

Asystole (Fig. 1.1) is the most common presenting rhythm in paediatric cardiac arrests (Sirbaugh *et al.*, 1999; Young & Seidel, 1999). It is the final common pathway of respiratory or circulatory failure (Zideman, 1997). Prolonged severe hypoxia and acidosis leads to progressive bradycardia and asystole (Advanced Life

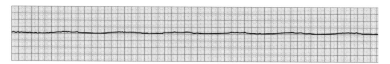

Fig. 1.1 Non-shockable rhythm: asystole.

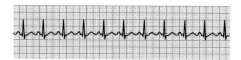

Fig. 1.2 Non-shockable rhythm: pulseless electrical activity.

Support Group, 2011). The most common cause is hypoxia, and the most effective treatment is to establish a clear airway and effective ventilation (Zideman, 1997).

Management of asystole is less commonly successful than when the rhythm is VF (Dieckmann & Vardis, 1995), but survival to discharge has been reported (Spearpoint, 2002).

Pulseless electrical activity

'Pulseless electrical activity' is a term used to signify the features of cardiac arrest associated with a normal (or near-normal) ECG (Fig. 1.2). The diagnosis is made on clinical grounds by the combination of the absence of a cardiac output with a ECG rhythm on the monitor that would normally be associated with a good cardiac output.

The causes of PEA can be classified into one of two broad categories:

- *Primary PEA* – there is failure of excitation contraction coupling in the cardiac myocytes resulting in a profound loss of cardiac output. Causes include hypoxia, poisoning, for example due to beta-blockers, calcium channel blockers or toxins, and electrolyte disturbance (hyperkalaemia or hypocalcaemia).
- *Secondary PEA* – there is a mechanical barrier to ventricular filling or ejection. Causes include hypovolaemia, cardiac tamponade and tension pneumothorax.

In all cases, treatment is directed towards the cause.

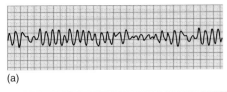

(a)

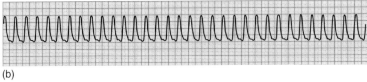

(b)

Fig. 1.3 Shockable rhythms: ventricular fibrillation (a) and pulseless ventricular tachycardia (b).

Ventricular fibrillation/pulseless ventricular tachycardia

VF/pulseless VT (Fig. 1.3) is uncommon in children (Zideman, 1997; Spearpoint, 2002). However, clinical situations when it may occur include after cardiac surgery or with cardiomyopathy, congenital heart disease, hypothermia or drug intoxication.

The ECG displays a bizarre irregular waveform, apparently random in both frequency and amplitude, which reflects disorganised electrical activity in the myocardium. This is an eminently treatable arrhythmia, but the only effective treatment is early defibrillation, and the likelihood of success is crucially time-dependent (Jevon, 2009).

Conditions for defibrillation are optimal for as little as 90 seconds after the onset of the rhythm, and the chances of success fall by about 10% with every minute that treatment is delayed (Waalewijn *et al.*, 2001). Untreated VF will inevitably deteriorate into asystole as myocardial energy reserves and oxygen are exhausted; successful cardiopulmonary resuscitation (CPR) at this late stage is almost impossible (Waalewijn *et al.*, 2001).

Importance of treating children differently from adults

Children are not small adults. Children are a diverse group of the population. They vary dramatically in weight, size, shape, intellectual ability and emotional responses.

At birth, a child is, on average, 3.5 kg, with a small respiratory and cardiovascular reserve and an immature immune system. At this stage, children are capable of limited movement, exhibit limited emotional responses and are dependent upon adults for their needs. Fourteen or more years later, at the other end of childhood, the adolescent is a 50 kg, 160 cm tall person who looks like an adult. Therefore, the competent management of the critically ill child, who may fall anywhere between these two extremes, requires a knowledge of these anatomical, physiological and emotional differences (Advanced Life Support Group, 2011).

Weight

The most dramatic changes in a child's weight occur during the first year of life: an average birth weight of 3.5 kg will increase to 10 kg by the child's first birthday. After this time, the weight increases more slowly until puberty. In paediatric resuscitation, most drugs and fluids are given per kilogram of body weight, so it is important to determine a child's weight as soon as possible during the treatment process.

The most accurate method is to weigh the child, but this may not always be possible, so in this situation a child's weight can be estimated in a number of methods. Examples of these are the Broselow tape, which relates the length of the child to the body weight, or centile charts that estimate weight against age. If a child's age is between 1 and 10 years, the most commonly used formula to determine weight (Resuscitation Council (UK), 2011) is:

$$\text{Weight (kg)} = \text{age (years)} + 4 \times 2$$

This formula is not, however, suitable for use in a child under 1 year of age: a term newborn infant averages 3.5 kg, and by 6 months the birth weight has usually doubled, trebling at 1 year.

Whichever method has been used to establish body weight, it is essential that healthcare professionals are familiar with and competent in its use.

Anatomical

A child's airway goes through many changes. In the younger child, the head is large and the neck short, which causes neck flexion and airway narrowing. The face and mandible are small, and the tongue is relatively large and can easily obstruct the airway. In addition, the floor of the mouth is easily compressible and can be obstructed by the positioning of the fingers during airway manoeuvres.

The anatomy of the airway itself also changes with age. Infants less than 6 moths of age are nose-breathers, and as upper respiratory tract infections are common in this age group, their airways are commonly obstructed by mucous secretions. In all young children, the epiglottis is horseshoe-shaped and the larynx high and anterior, making tracheal intubation much more difficult.

Physiological

There are many differences between the respiratory and cardiovascular systems of infants and those of adults (Tables 1.3–1.5). Infants have a greater metabolic rate and oxygen consumption, which is the reason for their increased respiratory rates. Stroke volume is also relatively small in infancy and increases with heart size. However, cardiac output is the product of stroke volume and heart rate so high cardiac outputs in infants and young children are achieved by rapid heart rates.

Table 1.3 Normal respiratory rate according to age

Age (years)	Respiratory rate (breaths/min)
<1	30–40
1–2	26–34
2–5	24–30
5–12	20–24
>12	12–20

Reproduced from Advanced Life Support Group (2011).

Table 1.4 Normal heart rate according to age

Age	Mean	Awake	Deep sleep
Newborn – 3 months	140	85–205	80–140
3 months – 2 years	130	100–180	75–160
2–10 years	80	60–140	60–90
>10 years	75	60–100	50–90

Reproduced from Advanced Life Support Group (2011).

Table 1.5 Normal blood pressure according to age

Age	Systolic blood pressure (mmHg)	
	Normal	Lower limit
0–1 month	>60	50–60
1–12 months	80	70
1–10 years	90 + 2 × age in years	70 + 2 × age in years
>10 years	120	90

Reproduced from Advanced Life Support Group (2011).

Immune function

At birth, the immune system is immature so babies are much more susceptible to illness.

Psychological

Children vary greatly in their intellectual ability and emotional response, and a knowledge of the child development is of great benefit to the practitioner. Infants and young children find it very difficult to communicate, and the importance of non-verbal communication and fear must be considered.

Cardiopulmonary resuscitation: standards for clinical practice and training

Cardiopulmonary Resuscitation: Standards for Clinical Practice and Training (Royal College of Anaesthetists *et al.*, 2008) is a joint statement from the Royal College of Anaesthetists, Royal College of Physicians of London, Intensive Care Society and Resuscitation Council (UK). It has been endorsed by a number of national bodies, including the Royal College of Nursing. The joint statement makes a numbers of recommendations relating to:

- The resuscitation committee
- The resuscitation officer
- Resuscitation training
- The prevention of cardiopulmonary arrest
- The resuscitation team

- Resuscitation in children, pregnancy and trauma
- Resuscitation equipment
- Decisions relating to CPR
- Patient transfer and post-resuscitation care
- Audit and reporting standards
- Research

Resuscitation committee

Each hospital should have a resuscitation committee that meets on a regular basis and is responsible for implementing operational policies relating to resuscitation practice and training. The chairperson should be a senior clinician who is actively involved in resuscitation. Membership of the committee should include:

- A physician
- A senior resuscitation officer
- An anaesthetist/intensivist
- A senior manager
- Representatives from appropriate departments, including paediatrics, based on local needs

The responsibilities of the resuscitation committee include:

- Advising on the composition and role of the resuscitation team
- Ensuring that resuscitation equipment and resuscitation drugs are available
- Ensuring the adequate provision of resuscitation training
- Ensuring that Resuscitation Council (UK) guidelines and standards for resuscitation are followed
- Updating resuscitation and anaphylaxis policies
- Recording and reporting clinical incidents related to resuscitation
- Auditing resuscitation attempts and Do Not Attempt Resuscitation (DNAR) orders

Resuscitation officer

Each hospital should have a resuscitation officer responsible for resuscitation training, ideally one for every 750 members of clinical staff. The resuscitation officer should possess a current

Resuscitation Council (UK) Advanced Life Support (ALS) certificate and should ideally be a Resuscitation Council (UK) ALS
Instructor. Adequate training facilities, training equipment and
secretarial support should be provided. Responsibilities of the
resuscitation officer include:

- Implementing Resuscitation Council (UK) guidelines and
  standards in resuscitation
- Providing adequate resuscitation training for relevant hospital
  personnel
- Ensuring that there are systems in place for checking and
  maintaining the resuscitation equipment
- Auditing resuscitation attempts following national guidelines
- Attending resuscitation attempts and providing feedback to
  team members
- Coordinating participation in resuscitation-related trials
- Keeping abreast of current resuscitation guidelines

Resuscitation training

Clinical staff should receive regular (at least annual) resuscitation
training appropriate to their level and expected clinical responsibilities. This should also be incorporated into the induction
programme for new staff. Where appropriate, this training should
include paediatric resuscitation training, incorporating the recognition and effective treatment of critical illness and providing
effective treatment to prevent cardiopulmonary arrest. Some
staff, for example members of the paediatric cardiac arrest team,
will require appropriate advanced resuscitation training, such as
a European Paediatric Life Support (EPLS) course or Advanced
Paediatric Life Support (APLS) course (see Chapter 15).

The resuscitation officer is responsible for organising and coordinating the training; a cascade system of training may be needed
to meet training demands, particularly in paediatric basic life
support. Help should be sought from other medical and nursing
specialties to provide specific training. See Chapter 15 for more
detailed information on resuscitation training.

Prevention of cardiopulmonary arrest

Systems should be place to identify patients who are critically ill
and therefore at risk of cardiopulmonary arrest (Royal College of

Anaesthetists *et al.*, 2008). Every hospital should have an early warning scoring system in place to identify these patients. Adverse clinical indicators or scores should elicit a response to alert expert help, for example the critical care outreach service or medical emergency team.

Each healthcare organization should have a patient observation chart that facilitates the regular measurement and recording of early warning scores. There should be a clear and specific policy that requires a clinical response to 'calling criteria' or early warning systems ('track and trigger'), including the specific responsibilities of senior medical and nursing staff (Royal College of Anaesthetists *et al.*, 2008).

Paediatric resuscitation team

The composition of the paediatric resuscitation team should be determined by the resuscitation committee. All staff who are involved with paediatric resuscitation should be encouraged to attend national paediatric courses such as the EPLS, APLS or Newborn Life Support course.

The resuscitation team should be alerted within 30 seconds of dialling 2222 (the recommended telephone number for contacting the switchboard following an in-hospital cardiac arrest) (National Patient Safety Agency, 2004). The system should be tested on a daily basis.

Resuscitation equipment

The resuscitation committee is responsible for advising on resuscitation equipment, which will largely be dependent upon local requirements and facilities. Ideally, it should be standardised throughout the hospital. The Resuscitation Council (UK) (2011) has made suggestions regarding resuscitation equipment for paediatric resuscitation, and these are discussed in detail in Chapter 2.

Do Not Attempt Resuscitation orders

Every hospital should have a DNAR policy, which should be based on national guidelines (BMA *et al.*, 2007). Only a minority of childhood deaths, such as those due to end-stage neoplastic disease, are expected and 'managed'. There should be timely discussions between the child, family and health carers to identify whether and in what manner resuscitation should be carried out to prevent unwanted and inappropriate resuscitation and interventions (Advanced Life Support Group, 2011).

Transfer of the child and post-resuscitation care

Complete recovery from a cardiac arrest is rarely immediate, and the return of spontaneous circulation is just the start, not the end, of the resuscitation attempt. The immediate post-resuscitation period is characterised by high dependency and clinical instability (Jevon, 2009), with most children requiring transfer to a paediatric intensive therapy unit. The principles of transfer of the child and post resuscitation care are discussed in Chapter 11.

Auditing and reporting standards

The resuscitation committee should ensure that all resuscitation attempts are audited. Acute NHS Trusts that are affiliated to the National Cardiac Arrest Audit (NCAA) initiative will submit data from paediatric resuscitation attempts to this audit. For further information, see Chapter 13.

To help ensure a high-quality resuscitation service, each hospital should audit:

- The resuscitation attempt, including outcomes
- The availability and use of resuscitation equipment
- The availability of emergency drugs
- DNAR orders
- Critical incidents that cause, or occur during, cardiopulmonary arrests
- Health and safety issues, including the cleaning and decontamination of resuscitation training manikins (following each training session)

Hospital management should be informed of any problems that arise, and the local clinical governance lead should support the resuscitation committee to rectify any deficiencies in the service.

Research

Healthcare practitioners interested in undertaking resuscitation-related research should be encouraged to do so. They should be advised to seek the advice and support of the local research ethics committee.

Summary

In this chapter, an overview of PALS has been provided. The causes of death in childhood have been discussed, together with the survival rates following paediatric resuscitation. The pathophysiology of paediatric cardiac arrests has been outlined, and the provision of a resuscitation service in hospital has been discussed.

References

Advanced Life Support Group (2011) *Advanced Paediatric Life Support*, 5th edn. Wiley Blackwell, Oxford.

American Academy of Pediatrics (2000) *Pediatric Education for Prehospital Professionals*. Jones & Bartlett, Sudbury, USA.

British Medical Association, Resuscitation Council (UK) & Royal College of Nursing (2007) *Decisions Relating to Cardiopulmonary Resuscitation. A Joint Statement from the British Medical Association, the Resuscitation*. BMA Resuscitation Council (UK) & RCN, London.

Dieckmann R, Vardis R (1995) High-dose epinephrine in pediatric out-of-hospital cardiopulmonary arrest. *Pediatrics*, **99**, 403–408.

Jevon, P. (2009) *Advanced Cardiac Life Support*, 2nd edn. Wiley Blackwell, Oxford.

Klitzener, T. (1995) Sudden cardiac death in children. *Circulation*, **82**, 629–632.

National Patient Safety Agency (2004) Establishing a Standard Crash Call Telephone Number in Hospitals. Retrieved from http://www.nrls.npsa.nhs.uk/resources/?EntryId45=59789 (accessed 3 June 2011).

Office for National Statistics (2009) *Child Mortality Statistics: Childhood, Infant and Perinatal, 2009*. Office for National Statistics, Newport, Gwent.

O'Rourke, P. (1986) Outcome of children who are apneic and pulseless in the emergency room. *Critical Care Medicine*, **14**, 466–468.

Resuscitation Council (UK) (2011) Suggested Equipment for the Management of Paediatric Cardiopulmonary Arrest (0–16 years) (Excluding

Resuscitation at Birth). Retrieved from: http://www.resus.org.uk (accessed 3 June 2011).

(Royal College of Anaesthetists, Royal College of Physicians of London, Intensive Care Society & Resuscitation Council (UK) (2008) *Cardiopulmonary Resuscitation: Standards for Clinical Practice and Training*. London: Authors.

Sirbaugh, P., Pepe, P., Shook, J. *et al.* (1999) A prospective, population-based study of the demographics, epidemiology, management, and outcome of out-of-hospital pediatric cardiopulmonary arrest. *Ann Emerg Med*, **33**, 174–184.

Spearpoint, K. (2002) National Audit of Paediatric Resuscitation (NAPR). Presentation at Resuscitation Council (UK) Instructor's Day, Birmingham, 11 April.

Stevenson, W.G. & Tedrow, U. (2010) Preventing ventricular tachycardia with catheter ablation. *Lancet*, **375**, 4–6.

Waalewijn, R., de Vos, R., Tijssen, J. & Koster, R. (2001) Survival models for out-of-hospital cardiopulmonary resuscitation from the perspectives of the bystander, the first responder and the paramedic. *Resuscitation*, **51**, 113–122.

Young, K. & Seidel, J. (1999) Pediatric cardiopulmonary resuscitation: a collective review. *Annals of Emergency Medicine*, **33**, 195–205.

Zaritsky, A., Nadkarni, V., Getson, P. & Kuehl, K. (1987) CPR in children. *Annals of Emergency Medicine*, **16**, 1107–1111.

Zideman, D. (1997) Paediatric resuscitation. In *Cardiopulmonary Resuscitation* (eds D. Skinner & R. Vincent), 2nd edn. Oxford University Press, Oxford.

Zideman, D. & Spearpoint, K. (1999) Resuscitation in infants and children. In *ABC of Resuscitation* (ed. M. Colquhoun), 4th edn. BMJ Books, London.

Chapter 2

Resuscitation Equipment for Paediatric Resuscitation

Introduction

A speedy response is essential in the event of a paediatric cardiac arrest. The Royal College of Anaesthetists, Royal College of Physicians of London, Intensive Care Society and Resuscitation Council (UK) (2004) have made recommendations on what resuscitation equipment (and medications) should be available for a paediatric arrest. Procedures should be in place to ensure that all the essential equipment is immediately available, accessible and in good working order.

A carefully set out and fully stocked cardiac arrest trolley is paramount. Ideally, the equipment used for paediatric cardiopulmonary resuscitation (including defibrillators) and the layout of equipment and drugs on resuscitation trolleys should be standardised throughout an institution (Royal College of Anaesthetists *et al.*, 2004).

The aim of this chapter is to understand what resuscitation equipment is required for paediatric resuscitation.

Learning objectives

At the end of this chapter, the reader will be able to:

- List the resuscitation equipment required for paediatric resuscitation
- List the aids available to estimate paediatric drug doses and equipment sizes
- Discuss the routine checking of resuscitation equipment
- Discuss the checking of resuscitation equipment following use

Paediatric Advanced Life Support: A Practical Guide for Nurses, Second Edition.
Phil Jevon.
© 2012 Phil Jevon. Published 2012 by Blackwell Publishing Ltd.

Resuscitation equipment required for paediatric resuscitation

The choice of paediatric resuscitation equipment should be defined by the resuscitation committee, depending upon on the anticipated workload, the availability of equipment from nearby departments and specialised local requirements (Royal College of Anaesthetists *et al.*, 2004). The Resuscitation Council UK (2011) suggests that the following resuscitation equipment and medications should be available to manage a paediatric arrest. All items should be latex-free, and all intravenous equipment should be Luer-locking.

Airway and breathing equipment

- Non-rebreathing oxygen masks – paediatric and adult
- Pocket masks – paediatric and adult ± face shields
- Oropharangeal airways – sizes 00, 0, 1, 2, 3 and 4
- Self-inflating bag-valve-mask systems:
  - Paediatric with pressure relief valve and reservoir
  - Adult with reservoir
- Face masks – sizes 00, 0/1, 2, 3 and 4
- Soft suction catheters – sizes 6, 8, 10, 12, 14
- Rigid-bore suction catheters – mini and adult
- Portable suction – battery or hand-operated
- Tracheal tubes – uncuffed sizes 2.5–6, cuffed sizes 6, 7 and 8
- Laryngoscopes
- Laryngoscope blades – straight sizes 0 and 1, curved sizes 2, 3 and 4
- Stethoscope
- $ETCO_2$ detectors (easily available)
- Nasogastric tubes – sizes 6, 8, 10 and 12
- Tracheal stylets – small and medium
- Gum elastic bougies – 5 ch and 10 ch
- Magill forceps – paediatric and adult
- Lubricating gel
- Elastoplast/hypofix/cotton tape
- Scissors
- Spare bulbs and batteries
- Oxygen cylinder – with tubing

Circulation equipment

- Alcohol skin preparation wipes
- Cannulae – 14, 16, 18, 20, 22 and 24 gauge
- Intraosseous needles
- Syringes – 1, 2, 5, 10, 20 and 50 mL
- Selection of needles
- Saline ampoules – 10 mL
- Water ampoules – 10 mL
- Extension set with T connectors, three-way taps and bungs
- Gauze
- Tape and dressing for cannulas
- Intravenous administration sets (burette and non-burrette)
- Blood bottles (easily available):
  - Full blood count, urea and electrolytes and C-reactive protein
  - Glucose
  - Blood cultures
  - Virology
  - Clotting
  - Crossmatch
  - Group and save
  - Toxicology
  - Arterial blood gas and capillary tubes
- Fluids:
  - Colloid solution
  - 0.9% sodium chloride or balanced salt solution
  - 10% dextrose
- Drugs
  - 1:10 000 adrenaline
  - 1:1000 adrenaline
  - Amiodarone + 5% dextrose
  - Lignocaine
  - Sodium bicarbonate 8.4%
  - Calcium chloride 10%
- Other readily available drugs (for use for paediatric emergencies):
  - Adenosine
  - Alprostidil
  - Atropine
  - Salbutamol
  - Ipratroprium

 – Diazepam/lorazepam
 – Midazolam
 – Morphine
 – Rapid sequence induction agents
 – Magnesium
 – Naloxone

(Source: Resuscitation Council (UK), 2011)

Additional items

- Paediatric resuscitation chart or tape (or similar)
- ECG electrodes
- Defibrillation gel pads
- Clock
- Gloves, goggles and aprons
- A sliding sheet or similar device for safer handling
- Pulse oximeter or capnography device

(Source: Royal College of Anaesthetists *et al.*, 2004; Resuscitation Council (UK), 2011)

The resuscitation equipment should be stored on a standard cardiac arrest trolley (Fig. 2.1), which should be spacious, sturdy, easily accessible and mobile. Every trolley should be identically stocked to avoid confusion. A defibrillator (with paediatric paddles) should also be immediately available.

Although piped or wall oxygen and suction should always be used when available, portable suction devices and oxygen should still be at hand either on or adjacent to the cardiac arrest trolley. Other items that the cardiac arrest team should have immediate access to include a stethoscope, an ECG machine, a blood pressure measuring device, a pulse oximeter, blood gas syringes and a device for verifying correct tracheal tube placement, e.g. an oesophageal detector device.

Aids to estimating paediatric drug doses and equipment sizes

Estimating drug doses and equipment sizes is important when managing a paediatric cardiac arrest. Several aids are currently available that help with these calculations, including the Walsall Paediatric Resuscitation Chart, the Oakley Chart and the

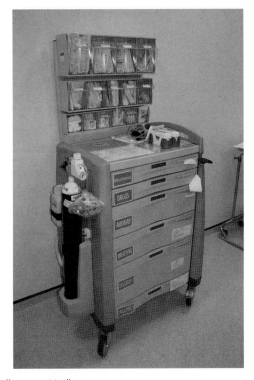

Fig. 2.1 Cardiac arrest trolley.

Broselow/Hinkle Paediatric Emergency System. It is important to become familiar with one specific system.

Walsall Paediatric Resuscitation Chart

The Walsall Paediatric Resuscitation Chart (Fig. 2.2) has been designed based on recommendations by Burke and Bowden (1993). A recent study has favoured the simple and clear approach that this chart has adopted, with all the drug doses recommended in millilitres using standard concentrations.

Oakley chart

The Oakley chart was first proposed in 1988 (Oakley, 1988). It was recognised at that time that a simple, versatile and readily available reference chart was required for paediatric resuscitation because of the variation in size of infants and children and the

Walsall Healthcare NHS
NHS Trust

WALSALL PAEDIATRIC RESUSCITATION CHART

NB All drug doses are in millilitres (mls), intravenous or intraosseous unless otherwise stated

Age	Months										
	3	6	1	2	3	4	5	6	8	10	12
Weight (Kg)	5	7	10	12	14	16	18	20	26	30	38
Adrenaline 1:10 000	0.5	0.7	1	1.2	1.4	1.6	1.8	2	2.6	3	3.8
Amiodarone 50mg/ml	0.5	0.7	1	1.2	1.4	1.6	1.8	2	2.6	3	3.8
Atropine 1mg/10mls	1	1.4	2	2.4	2.8	3.2	3.6	4	5.2	6	6
Calcium Chloride 10%	1	1.4	2	2.4	2.8	3.2	3.6	4	5.2	6	7.6
Fluid Bolus 0.9% Saline	100	140	200	240	280	320	360	400	520	600	760
Glucose 10%	10	14	20	24	28	32	36	40	52	60	76
Sodium bicarbonate 8.4%	5	7	10	12	14	16	18	20	26	30	38
Defibrillation (Joules)	20	30	40	50	60	60	70	80	100	120	150
ET tube (cuffed) (ID: mm)	3	3	3.5	4	4-4.5	4.5	4.5-5	5	6-6.5	7	7-7.5
ETtube (uncuffed) (ID: mm)	3.5	3.5	4	4.5	4.5-5	5	5-5.5	5.5			
ET tube (length cm)	9	10	12	13	13	14	15	15	16	17	18

References
Burke D, Bowden D (1993) Modified Paediatric Chart. BMJ 306:1096-82
Jevon P (2011) Advanced Paediatric Life Support 2nd Edition Wiley Blackwell, Oxford
Resuscitation Council UK (2011) European Paediatric Life Support 2nd Edition Resuscitation Council UK, London
Resuscitation Council UK (2011) Paediatric Emergency Treatment Chart www.resus.org.uk accessed 20/05/11
UK-WHO (2009) Boys UK-WHO Growth Chart 0-4 Years http://www.rcpch.ac.uk/Research/UK-WHO-Growth-Charts accessed 14/10/09
Acknowledgements
Chart revised by P Jevon, with help from D Burke, N Rashid, D Bowden, R Joshi, A Ismail, S Northcliffe, D Ferdinand, I Darwood, K Berry & G Pearson
Body weights – averaged on lean body weights taken as 50th Centile value for boys & girls
This poster has been produced with a grant from UCB Pharma.
WALSALL HEALTHCARE NHS TRUST 05/11

Fig. 2.2

comparative infrequency of paediatric cardiopulmonary arrests. The chart has now been revised.

Broselow/Hinkle Paediatric Emergency System

The Broselow/Hinkle Paediatric Emergency System provides a fast, accurate method for selecting emergency equipment and drug doses. First, the child's length is measured and assigned one of the seven colour ranges. A coordinated colour pack is taken from the Broselow/Hinkle system. The full system comprises a manual resuscitation system, intubation modules, oxygen delivery modules, intravenous delivery modules, intraosseous access modules and blood pressure cuffs.

Routine checking of resuscitation equipment

Resuscitation equipment should be checked daily by each ward or department with responsibility for the resuscitation trolley (Royal College of Anaesthetists *et al.*, 2004).

A system for daily documented checks of the equipment inventory should be in place. Some cardiac arrest trolleys can be 'sealed' with a numbered seal after being checked. Once the contents have been checked, the trolley can then be sealed and the seal number documented by the person who has checked the trolley. The advantage of this system is that an unbroken seal, together with the same seal number last recorded, signifies that the trolley has not been opened since it was last checked and sealed. The equipment inventory should therefore be complete. A broken seal or an unrecorded seal number suggests the inventory may not be complete, and a complete check is then required. The seal can easily be broken if the trolley needs to be opened.

Expiry dates should be checked for, for example, drugs, fluids, ECG electrodes and defibrillation pads. Laryngoscopes, including batteries and bulbs, should also be checked to ensure good working order. Each self-inflating bag should be checked to ensure that there are no leaks and that the rim of the face mask is adequately inflated.

The defibrillator should be checked on a daily basis following the manufacturer's recommendations. This usually will involve charging up and discharging the shock into the defibrillator. It is recommended that advice is sought from a member of the electro-biomedical engineers department (EBME) or from the manufacturer's representative regarding how to undertake this. In addition, most defibrillators need to be plugged into the mains to ensure that the battery is fully charged in case it needs to be used.

Manufacturers usually recommend that ECG electrodes should be stored in their original packaging until immediately prior to use. However, the policy at some hospitals is to leave them attached to the defibrillator leads. They should therefore be checked to ensure that the gel is moist and not dry. If the electrodes are dry, they should be replaced.

All mechanical equipment, e.g. defibrillator and suction machine, should be inspected and serviced on a regular basis by the EBME department following the manufacturer's recommendations.

Checking resuscitation equipment following use

Checking of resuscitation equipment following use should be a specifically delegated responsibility. As well as the routine checks identified above, any disposable equipment used should be replaced, and reusable equipment, e.g. the self-inflating bag, cleaned following local infection control procedures and the manufacturer's recommendations. Any difficulties with equipment encountered during resuscitation should be documented and reported to the relevant personnel.

Summary

This chapter has made suggestions for what resuscitation equipment should be immediately available in the event of a paediatric cardiac arrest. Suggestions have also been made regarding the storage, checking and maintenance of this equipment. Aids to calculating drug doses and equipment sizes for paediatric resuscitation have also been outlined.

References

Burke, D. & Bowden, D. (1993) Modified paediatric resuscitation chart. *BMJ*, **306**, 1096–1098.

Oakley, P. (1988) Inaccuracy and delay in decision making in paediatric resuscitation and a proposed reference chart to reduce error. *BMJ*, **297**, 817–819.

Resuscitation Council (UK) (2011) Suggested Equipment for the Management of Paediatric Cardiopulmonary Arrest (0–16 years) (excluding resuscitation at birth). Retrieved from http://www.resus.org.uk (accessed 3 June 2011).

Royal College of Anaesthetists, Royal College of Physicians of London, Intensive Care Society and Resuscitation Council (UK) (2004) *Cardiopulmonary Resuscitation: Standards for Clinical Practice and Training*. Resuscitation Council (UK), London.

Chapter 3

Recognition of the Seriously Ill Child

Jayne Breakwell

Introduction

Cardiorespiratory arrest in children is usually due to hypoxia, reflecting the end of the body's ability to compensate for the effects of underlying illness or injury (Resuscitation Council (UK), 2011).

Using the structured ABCDE approach (Box 3.1) helps to ensure that potentially life-threatening problems are identified and dealt with in order of priority: the early recognition and effective management of respiratory and/or circulatory failure will hopefully prevent deterioration to cardiorespiratory arrest (Resuscitation Council (UK), 2011).

The aim of this chapter is to understand the recognition of the seriously ill child.

Learning objectives

At the end of this chapter, the reader will be able to:

- Discuss the aetiology of cardiorespiratory arrests in children
- Outline the ABCDE approach

Paediatric Advanced Life Support: A Practical Guide for Nurses, Second Edition.
Phil Jevon.
© 2012 Phil Jevon. Published 2012 by Blackwell Publishing Ltd.

> **Box 3.1** ABCDE approach to assess and treat the critically ill child (Resuscitation Council (UK), 2011)
>
> - Airway
> - Breathing
> - Circulation
> - Disability
> - Exposure

Aetiology of cardiorespiratory arrests in children

The aetiology of cardiorespiratory arrest in children usually differs greatly from that in adults, owing to the anatomical, physiological and pathological differences that occur throughout childhood.

In adults, cardiorespiratory arrests are commonly caused by cardiac arrhythmias relating to underlying ischaemic heart disease; such arrests are an acute event and can occur without warning. In children, however, cardiorespiratory arrest is rarely a sudden event, but a progressive deterioration as respiratory and circulatory failure worsen (Fig. 3.1). In children, cardiorespiratory arrest is usually caused by hypoxia, reflecting the end of the body's ability to compensate for the effects of underlying illness or injury (Resuscitation Council (UK), 2011). Some of the causes of respiratory failure and circulatory failure are listed in Box 3.2.

ABCDE approach

The ABCDE approach (see Box 3.1) can, as in adults, be used when assessing and treating a critically ill child; the underlying principles of assessment, initial management and ongoing reassessment are the same. The general principles are as follows:

- Observe the child generally to determine the overall level of illness (i.e. does the child look seriously unwell?; is he or she interacting with the parents?).
- Speak to the child and assess the appropriateness of the response; ask the parents about the child's 'usual' behaviour.
- If the child is unconscious and unresponsive to your voice, administer tactile stimulation (gently shake the arm or leg). If the child responds by speaking or crying, this indicates that

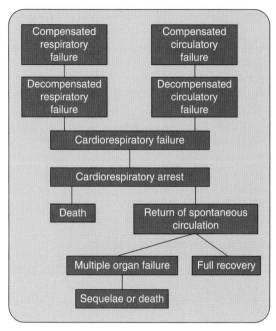

Fig. 3.1 Pathways leading to cardiopulmonary arrest in children (Resuscitation Council (UK) 2011).

Box 3.2 Causes of respiratory and circulatory failure in children (Advanced Life Support Group, 2011) – note that this is not an exhaustive list

Respiratory failure

- Asthma
- Bronchiolitis
- Foreign body airway obstruction
- Medications
- Head injury
- Anaphylaxis
- Seizures

Circulatory failure

- Severe diarrhoea and vomiting
- Meningococcal septicaemia
- Anaphylaxis
- Trauma and blood loss

there is a patent airway, that the child is breathing and that the brain is perfused. Regardless of the child's response to initial stimulation, move on rapidly to a full ABCDE assessment.

- Appropriate high-flow oxygen delivery should be immediately commenced.
- Vital sign monitoring should be requested early.
- Circulatory access should be achieved as soon as possible. Bloods for laboratory investigations and a bedside blood glucose level should be obtained.
- Ensure personal safety

(Source: Advanced Life Support Group, 2011; Resuscitation Council (UK), 2011)

Initial approach to the child

- Ensure that it is safe to approach the child. Check the environment and remove any hazards.
- On approaching the child, and before touching him or her, rapidly look around for any clues to what may have caused the emergency as this may influence the way the child is managed (e.g. it may arouse suspicion of a head or neck injury).
- Determine the child's responsiveness. An appropriate way of doing this is by calling the child's name and telling them to 'Wake up!' For an infant, it is appropriate to 'flick' the feet or pick the infant up if no trauma is suspected. A normal response implies that the child has a patent airway, is breathing and has cerebral perfusion. An inappropriate response or no response indicates that the child may be critically ill and that help needs to be summoned immediately.

Assessment of the airway

If the child is talking or crying, there will be a patent airway. In a conscious child, it is important to establish airway patency – is the airway at risk or obstructed? Airway obstruction can be partial or complete. The airway may be restricted by mucous or vomit, and simple actions such as repositioning or suction may be required. A foreign body may be present, and in unconscious children the tongue may fall backwards and occlude the airway. Airway obstruction may be demonstrated by difficulty in breathing and /or increased respiratory rate; if the obstruction is partial, there may be gurgling or stridor. When assessing airway patency, it is important to note that chest movement does not guarantee that the airway is clear.

Causes of airway obstruction include:

- A foreign body
- The tongue
- Secretions – vomit/blood
- Respiratory tract infections
- An altered level of consciousness
- Pharyngeal swelling
- Epiglottitis
- Laryngospasm or bronchospasm
- Trauma – to the face or throat
- Congenital abnormality

(Source: Advanced Life Support Group, 2011; Resuscitation Council (UK), 2011)

The airway can usually be opened using the head tilt–chin lift manoeuvre. Place one hand on the child's forehead and gently tilt the head back; in the infant (under 1 year of age), this is the neutral position, and for the child, this is the 'sniffing the morning air' position with some extension of the head and neck required. If this position is not possible or any trauma is suspected, a jaw thrust manoeuvre can be performed. This is achieved by placing two or three fingers under the angle of the mandible bilaterally and lifting the jaw upwards.

In children with airway obstruction, it is important to deliver supplemental oxygen as soon as possible to minimize the effects of hypoxia. If there is a reduced level of consciousness, airway compromise must be assumed – the familiar 'look, listen and feel' approach can easily detect if an airway is obstructed:

- *Look* – for chest and abdominal movements. If the airway is obstructed, paradoxical chest movements (see-saw respirations) and the use of accessory muscles can be seen.
- *Listen* – for breathing. Normal respirations are quiet, partially obstructed breathing is usually noisy, and complete obstruction will be silent.
- *Feel* – for signs of airway obstruction. Place your face in front of the child's mouth to determine whether there is any movement of air.

Treatment of airway obstruction

Once airway obstruction has been identified, treat it appropriately. Simple methods such as suctioning, airway positioning or insertion of an oropharyngeal or nasopharyngeal airway are often very effective. As described earlier, administer high–flow oxygen as soon as possible.

Assessment of breathing

Once the airway is open, it is important to assess for effective, spontaneous breathing. Appropriate management of the airway and breathing is the priority in all seriously ill children. This is also achieved by the 'look, listen and feel' approach.

Look

Look for general signs of respiratory distress. Look at the respiratory rate, the work of breathing and the tidal volume. Is there tachypnoea, central cyanosis, chest expansion or any use of accessory muscles? In children, recognition of respiratory failure is based on a full assessment of respiratory effort and efficacy, and the effects of this inadequacy on the major organs (Resuscitation Council (UK), 2011).

Tachypnoea is usually the first sign of respiratory insufficiency (Smith, 2003). As discussed earlier, normal respiratory ranges vary with age, and it is important to consider this (see Table 1.3). But it is important to remember that fever, pain and anxiety will also alter the respiratory rate; therefore, it is more important to monitor the trend in the rate rather than rely on absolute values (Resuscitation Council (UK), 2011).

Recession – sternal, subcostal or intercostal – is common in the sick child and shows the effort of breathing. The degree of recession provides an indication of the severity of the respiratory distress. Infants and younger children can exhibit significant recession with relatively mild-to-moderate respiratory compromise owing to their highly compliant chest wall. However, in children over approximately 5 years of age, recession is a sign of significant respiratory compromise (Resuscitation Council (UK), 2011).

The use of accessory muscles is also a common sign when the work of breathing is increased. The sternocleidomastoid muscle in the neck is often used as an accessory respiratory muscle (Resuscitation Council (UK), 2011). In infants, this can cause the head to move up and down with each breath, a sign known as 'head-bobbing'.

Another common breathing pattern seen in severe respiratory distress is 'see-saw' breathing, which is the paradoxical movement of the abdomen during inspiration. This, however, is a very inefficient pattern of respiration because the tidal volume is greatly reduced. Nostril flaring can also be seen in infants and young children.

The depth of breathing should also be assessed. Ascertain whether chest movement is equal on both sides: unilateral chest movement may be a sign of pneumothorax, pneumonia or pleural effusion (Smith, 2003).

Children in respiratory compromise will usually adopt a position that aids their respiratory capacity. This position must be supported to maximize their comfort and prevent further upset that might result in further deterioration.

The degree of increased work of breathing generally provides clinical evidence of the severity of respiratory insufficiency, but there are exceptions to this (Resuscitation Council (UK), 2011):

- *Exhaustion* – children who have had severe respiratory compromise for some time may have progressed to decompensation and no longer show signs of increased work of breathing. Exhaustion is a preterminal event.
- *Neuromuscular disease* – muscular dystrophy, for example, may be present.
- *Central respiratory depression* – reduced respiratory drive, e.g. with encephalopathy or medications such as morphine, results in respiratory inadequacy.

Pulse oximetry should be used on any child showing signs of respiratory distress who is at risk of respiratory failure. An arterial oxygen saturation (Sao_2) of less than 90% in air or <95% in supplemental oxygen indicates respiratory failure. It should be noted that Sao_2 measurements are unreliable when a child has a poor peripheral circulation. In addition, when Sao_2 is below 70%, pulse oximetry is inaccurate.

Listen

Listen to the child's breath sounds a short distance from the face. Normal breathing is quiet. Noisy breathing indicates the presence of airway obstruction (Advanced Life Support Group, 2011; Resuscitation Council (UK), 2011):

- *Stridor* – associated with partial upper airway obstruction. Wheezing is generally an expiratory noise.
- *Wheeze* – may be heard audibly or on chest auscultation with a stethoscope. It indicates narrowing of the lower airways, e.g. bronchospasm.
- *Grunting* – is mainly heard in young babies, but can occur in small children. It is the result of exhaling against a partially closed glottis, and is an attempt to generate a positive end-expiratory pressure, thus preventing airway collapse at the end of expiration. Grunting is usually associated with 'stiff' lungs and is an indication of severe respiratory compromise.

If possible, the chest should be auscultated. Air entry should be heard in all areas of the lungs. The depth and equality of breath sounds on both sides of the chest should be evaluated. Any additional sounds, e.g. a crackle or wheeze, should be noted, and it is often useful to compare one side of the chest with the other. A silent chest indicates a dangerously reduced tidal volume and is an ominous sign.

Feel
If possible, palpate and percuss the chest wall. Palpation may identify deformities, surgical emphysema or crepitus (suggesting pneumothorax until proven otherwise) (Smith, 2003). Percussion of the chest wall can demonstrate areas of collapse (dullness) or hyperresonance (e.g. in pneumothorax).

Respiratory compromise also affects other systems of the body, including heart rate, skin perfusion and level of consciousness.

Management of respiratory compromise
The treatment of breathing problems depends on achieving a patent airway and an effective delivery of oxygen. This will vary with the child's clinical condition and age. Children who do have adequate spontaneous breathing should have high-flow oxygen delivered in a manner that is non-threatening and best tolerated by them, e.g. from a non-rebreathing face mask or nasal cannula.

When breathing is inadequate (or absent), high-flow oxygen should be delivered by ventilation with a bag-valve-mask system.

In situations where the child is exhausted and is likely to require ongoing respiratory support (or is in a state of imminent cardiorespiratory arrest), tracheal intubation may be indicated (Resuscitation Council (UK), 2011).

Assessment of circulation

Appropriate management of the airway and breathing is the priority in all sick children and should be initiated before assessing the circulatory status.

Circulatory failure is the clinical state in which the flow of blood (and the associated delivery of nutrients, e.g. oxygen and glucose) to the body tissues is inadequate to meet the metabolic demand (Resuscitation Council (UK), 2011). In children, the majority of cases of circulatory failure result from hypovolaemia, sepsis or anaphylaxis. Other uncommon causes include obstruction of blood flow, e.g. tension pneumothorax, or anaemia or carbon monoxide poisoning, in which the oxygen-carrying capacity of the blood is reduced.

Children initially compensate for reduced tissue perfusion, so it is essential to promptly recognize and treat any child with compensated circulatory failure to prevent deterioration to a decompensated state. The familiar 'look, listen and feel' approach can be used to assess the circulation.

Look

Look at the skin temperature and colour, heart rate, capillary refill time and conscious level. The skin of a healthy child is pink and warm to the touch. Signs of cardiovascular compromise include cool, pale, mottled peripheries. Demarcation lines are also seen in very sick children; these indicate peripheral vasoconstriction and decreased perfusion, which leaves a line between the warm and the cold skin.

Measure the capillary refill time (CRT). A normal CRT is less than 2 seconds, but this is prolonged when there is reduced skin perfusion. In children with pyrexia and those who have cool peripheries, a central CRT reading (e.g. the chest or forehead) is much more reliable.

Also look for other signs of a poor cardiac output, e.g. a reduced level of consciousness or poor urinary output – the parents of young children will be very aware how many wet nappies their child has had that day. A urine output below 2 mL/ kg per hour in infants and below 1 mL/kg per hour in children indicates inadequate renal perfusion (Resuscitation Council (UK), 2011).

Listen
Measure the child's blood pressure. In most forms of shock, a child's blood pressure can be maintained within the normal range (Table 1.1) for a period of time (except in sepsis and anaphylaxis); once compensation is no longer possible, hypotension occurs (Resuscitation Council (UK), 2011).

In hypovolaemia, hypotension occurs only once about 40% of the child's circulatory volume has been lost. It is therefore important to recognise when the child is in compensated circulatory failure and manage the condition effectively early on before decompensation occurs (Resuscitation Council (UK), 2011).

Hypotension is a sign of physiological decompensation and indicates imminent cardiorespiratory arrest.

Feel
Feel the central pulse. The heart rate will initially rise to maintain cardiac output. Heart rate varies with age (see Table 1.4), but is also altered by fever, pain and anxiety, so other signs of circulatory function must also be observed. When the heart rate is unable to maintain tissue perfusion, the tissue hypoxia and acidosis result in bradycardia, and the presence of bradycardia is a preterminal sign.

The pulse volume gives a subjective indication of stroke volume – is the pulse strong or weak, thready or bounding, or is there a difference when comparing the central and peripheral pulses? In fact, is a pulse present at all?

Circulatory compromise also affects other systems of the body including respiratory function and level of consciousness.

Management of circulatory compromise
The treatment of circulatory problems is dependent on achieving a patent airway and effectively managing ventilation with the delivery of high-flow oxygen before turning the attention to circulatory procedures (Resuscitation Council (UK), 2011). Immediate life-threatening causes of circulatory failure must be sought and urgently treated.

Ideally, two large-bore vascular cannulas should be inserted as soon as possible. Intraosseous access may be indicated (see Chapter 8); this route can be used to deliver all resuscitation fluids, medications and blood-derived products.

Unless contraindicated (e.g. in cardiac failure), volume replacement should be initiated as soon as possible. A 20 mL/kg bolus of crystalloid solution, usually 0.9% saline, should be given as soon and as quickly as possible. The child's circulatory status should then be reassessed, and if signs of failure are still present, this should be repeated. A further infusion, making three in total, is also permitted if required while the underlying cause is sought. If the cause of the circulatory failure is identified as haemorrhage, blood products must be considered.

Glucose-containing solutions should never be used for volume replacement as they can be dangerous, causing hyponatraemia and hyperglycaemia (Resuscitation Council (UK), 2011).

Assessment of disability

Causes of altered levels of consciousness include hypoxia, hypoglycaemia and medications, so it is very important to:

- Review the airway, breathing and circulation to exclude anything previously missed
- Check the medication(s) already received if a drug-induced cause is suspected
- Undertake a bedside glucose measurement to exclude hypoglycaemia

A rapid assessment of conscious level can be carried out by using the AVPU scale:

- A – ALERT
- V – responds to VOICE
- P – responds to PAIN
- U – UNRESPONSIVE to painful stimuli

(Resuscitation Council 2011)

The Glasgow Coma Scale is another scale commonly used to assess level of consciousness; a child who is unresponsive to painful stimuli has an equivalent Glasgow Coma Scale score of 8 or less.

Interaction is also a good sign of disability. How is the child interacting with the parents and surroundings? It a worrying sign to see a young child lying very still and letting staff perform examinations and investigations on him or her.

Look at a child's posture. Is the infant floppy, or the young child drowsy? Is the child stiff, which may be the sign of a serious brain dysfunction?

Look at the pupillary reactions, and their size, equality and reaction to light. Are reactions brisk or sluggish?

Management of altered conscious level

The first priority is to reassess the airway, breathing and circulation to make sure that nothing has recurred or been missed. If hypoglycaemia is confirmed, administer glucose to correct it. This may be oral glucose if the child can tolerate it, or otherwise intravenous glucose. If a drug-induced alteration in level of consciousness is suspected and the effects are reversible, administer the antidote if it is available. It may be necessary to nurse the child in the lateral or the recovery position.

Exposure

Full exposure of the child is necessary in order to undertake a thorough examination and ensure that important details are not overlooked (Smith, 2003). Appropriate measures to minimise heat loss (especially in infants) and respect dignity must be adopted at all times.

Control any bleeding found, and reconsider fluid management as directed by fluid loss.

Look for evidence of blood loss, skin lesions, wounds and rashes – blanching or petechial. Direct treatment towards any rashes found; for example, a petechial rash is a sign of meningococcal septicaemia and needs antibiotics.

Are there bruises? Investigate any bruises for signs of malignancy, e.g. leukaemia, or non-accidental injury; the latter need referral to the safeguarding team for further investigation.

Check the child's core temperature. Is he or she pyrexial or hypothermic? Consider appropriate temperature measures, such as antipyretics or blankets or warm fluids.

In addition:

- Undertake a full clinical history
- Review the child's case notes, observation chart and prescription chart
- Ensure that prescribed medications and fluids are being administered
- Review laboratory and, radiology results once these become available
- Consider the level of care the child requires – ward, high-dependency unit or paediatric intensive care
- Provide effective communication to the child and parents or carers at all times

Summary

Early recognition and treatment of the seriously ill child is paramount. The Resuscitation Council (UK) (2011) recommends the ABCDE approach to recognise and treat serious illness in children.

References

Advanced Life Support Group (2011) *Advanced Paediatric Life Support*, 5th edn. Wiley, Oxford.

Resuscitation Council (UK) (2011) *Paediatric Immediate Life Support*, 2nd edn. Resuscitation Council (UK), London.

Smith G (2003) *Alert: Acute Life-threatening Events Recognition and Treatment*, 2nd edn. Portsmouth, University of Portsmouth.

Chapter 4

Paediatric Basic Life Support

Introduction

The aetiology of cardiopulmonary arrests in infants and children differs from that in adults (Hazinski, 1995; Advanced Life Support Group, 2011). Such arrests are normally secondary to either respiratory or circulatory failure, and rarely result from a primary cardiac event. Respiratory failure is the most common cause (Resuscitation Council (UK), 2011).

The priorities and sequence of paediatric basic life support (BLS) therefore follow the principle that early effective oxygenation and ventilation must be established as quickly as possible (Kitamura *et al.*, 2010). Indeed, survival from cardiopulmonary arrest is dependent mainly upon the immediate provision of effective rescue ventilation (Friesen *et al.*, 1982).

BLS refers to maintaining an open airway and supporting breathing and circulation without the use of equipment other than a protective shield. In the hospital setting, the availability of additional personnel and equipment (particularly airway/ ventilation adjuncts) requires an adaption of the conventional BLS guidelines. However, healthcare professionals must still have a working knowledge of BLS in case they need to perform it outside their normal working environment.

For the purpose of paediatric BLS, an infant can be defined as being under 1 year of age, and a child as being between 1 year and puberty (formally confirming the onset of puberty is not necessary and is indeed appropriate). If the 'victim' is actually an

Paediatric Advanced Life Support: A Practical Guide for Nurses, Second Edition.
Phil Jevon.
© 2012 Phil Jevon. Published 2012 by Blackwell Publishing Ltd.

adult but the paediatric guidelines have been used, little harm will be caused because the aetiology of cardiac arrests in children and young adults is the same (Safranek *et al.*, 1992). Therefore, if the victim is judged to be a child, the paediatric resuscitation guidelines should be followed (Resuscitation Council (UK), 2011).

The aim of this chapter is to understand the principles of paediatric BLS.

Learning objectives

At the end of this chapter, the reader will be able to:

- Discuss the sequence of actions in BLS
- Outline the principles of basic airway management
- Describe two methods of ventilation
- Describe the correct procedure for chest compression
- Describe the recovery position
- Outline the management of foreign body airway obstruction
- Outline the principles of safer handling during cardiopulmonary resuscitation (CPR)

Sequence of actions in basic life support

The initial assessment and sequence of actions in paediatric BLS should follow the SSSABCR approach (Box 4.1). The Resuscitation Council's paediatric BLS algorithm (Fig 4.1) guides the practitioner through the sequence for paediatric BLS.

The sequence of paediatric BLS described in this chapter is aimed at those who have a duty of care to respond to paediatric

---

Box 4.1 Initial assessment and sequence of actions in paediatric BLS (Resuscitation Council (UK), 2011)

- **S**afe
- **S**timulate
- **S**hout for assistance
- **A**irway
- **B**reathing
- **C**irculation
- **R**eassess

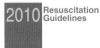 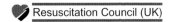

Paediatric Basic Life Support
(Healthcare professionals with a duty to respond)

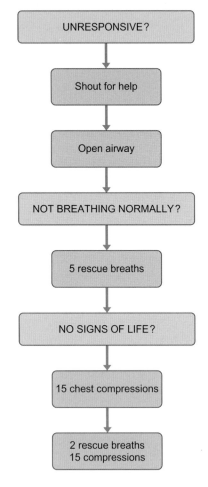

Call resuscitation team

Fig. 4.1 Resuscitation Council (UK) paediatric basic life support algorithm. Reproduced with kind permission of the Resuscitation Council (UK).

emergencies (usually healthcare practitioners). Those taught adult BLS who have no specific knowledge of paediatric resuscitation may use the adult sequence because the outcome will be worse if they do nothing. Non-specialists who need to be taught paediatric resuscitation techniques because they have responsibility for children (e.g. teachers, school nurses or lifeguards) should be taught that they should ideally modify the adult BLS sequence, i.e. perform five initial breaths followed by approximately 1 minute of CPR before going for help (Biarent *et* al., 2010).

This sequence to be followed in paediatric BLS will now be outlined.

Unresponsive?

Check whether the child is responsive:

- For an *infant*, gently rub the chest, blow on the face and tickle the feet (Fig. 4.2).
- With a *child*, gently shake the shoulders (exercise caution if cervical spinal injury is suspected) and ask loudly 'Are you all right?' (Fig. 4.3).

If there is a response, leave the infant or child in the position that he or she has been found, provided there is no chance of further danger. Establish the likely cause of the collapse and get help if necessary.

If there is *no response*, shout for help.

Shout for help

Shout for help. In some situations, pressing an emergency buzzer to alert colleagues will be appropriate. Then proceed to open the airway.

Open the airway

Turn the infant or child onto the back (unless full assessment is possible in the position the child has been found). Open the airway by tilting the head and lifting the chin (Fig. 4.4) (Roth *et al.*, 1998), remembering to exercise caution if cervical spine injury is suspected. Look in the mouth and remove any obvious obstruction. Then check whether the child is breathing normally.

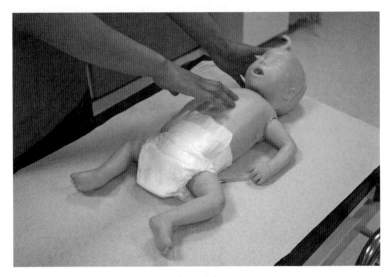

Fig. 4.2 Assessing responsiveness in an infant.

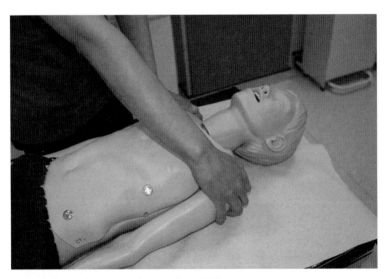

Fig. 4.3 Assessing responsiveness in a child.

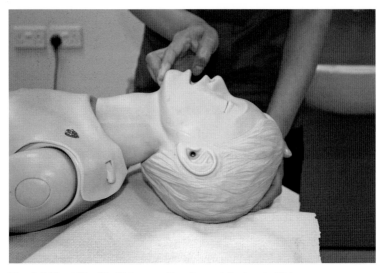

Fig. 4.4 Head tilt–chin lift to open the airway: infant and child.

Not breathing normally?

While maintaining an open airway, check for signs of normal breathing (more than an occasional gasp or weak attempts at breathing; Fig. 4.5) for up to 10 seconds:

- Look for a rise and fall of the chest and abdomen.
- Listen for airflow at the mouth and nose.
- Feel for airflow on your cheek.

It can sometimes be difficult to establish whether the infant/child is breathing (Ruppert *et al.*, 1999; Resuscitation Council (UK), 2011), and it is important to differentiate ineffective, gasping or obstructed respirations from effective respirations (Noc *et al.*, 1994; Poets *et al.*, 1999). If you are uncertain whether the infant/child is breathing, deliver rescue breaths (Biarent *et al.*, 2010).

If the infant/child *is breathing*, place him or her in the recovery position (exercise caution if there is a history of trauma), check for continued breathing and ensure that help is on the way.

If the infant/child *is not breathing*, send someone else for help and deliver rescue breaths.

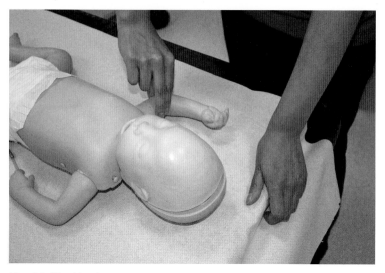

Fig. 4.5 Checking for signs of normal breathing.

Five rescue breaths

Deliver five initial rescue breaths. While delivering the rescue breaths, observe for any gag or cough response (signs of life – see below) to the rescue breaths. After delivering five initial rescue breaths, check for signs of life.

No signs of life?

Take no longer than 10 seconds to assess the child's circulation: look for signs of life such as movement, coughing or normal breathing.

If you are trained to do so, check for the pulse but for no longer than 10 seconds:

- *In an infant* – check for the brachial pulse as the short, chubby neck of an infant makes it difficult to check for the carotid pulse (Sarti *et al.*, 2005, 2006). The brachial pulse is located on the inside of the infant's upper arm, in between the elbow and the shoulder. Palpation of the femoral pulse is another option.

- *In a child* – check for the carotid pulse (Sarti *et al.*, 2005, 2006). First, locate the thyroid cartilage (Adam's apple) with two or three fingers from one hand (while maintaining the head tilt with the other). Then slide the fingers into the groove in between the trachea and the sternocleidomastoid muscles and gently palpate. Palpation of the femoral pulse is another option.

Healthcare practitioners struggle reliably to determine within 10 seconds the presence or absence of a pulse in infants and children (Tibballs & Weeranatna, 2010; Tibballs *et al.*, 2010), hence why it is also important to look for signs of life.

If there *are signs of life*, continue the rescue breaths at a rate of 20 per minute if necessary until the child begins to breath normally.

If there are *no signs of life*, deliver 15 chest compressions (unless the practitioner can definitely, within 10 seconds, feel a pulse of over 60 beats per minute).

Fifteen chest compressions

Perform 15 chest compressions at a rate of at least 100 per minute (but not over 120 per minute).

Two rescue breaths, 15 chest compressions

Combine chest compressions with rescue breaths in a ratio of 15:2 (15 chest compressions to 2 rescue breaths).

When to get help

If there is *more than one rescuer*, one should start CPR while the other gets help.

If there is just a *single rescuer*, he or she should perform CPR for 1 minute before getting help. (It may be possible to carry an infant or small child while simultaneously performing CPR and getting help.)

Note that the only exception to performing 1 minute of CPR before going for help is when the child has a sudden collapse witnessed by the practitioner: as the cardiac arrest is likely to be caused by an arrhythmia and the child may need defibrillation, it is important to seek help immediately (Biarent *et al.*, 2010).

Principles of basic airway management

The airway in an unconscious child can easily become obstructed by a combination of flexion of the neck, relaxation of the jaw, displacement of the tongue against the posterior wall of the pharynx and collapse of the hypopharynx (Hudgel & Hendricks, 1988; Abernethy *et al.*, 1990). In some cases, just opening the airway may revive the child.

The airway can be opened by tilting the head and lifting the chin. This will help to open the airway and bring the tongue forward from the posterior wall of the pharynx (the tongue being most common cause of airway obstruction in an unconscious child; Ruben *et al.*, 1961). The neutral position in an infant and the 'sniffing the morning air' position in a child are recommended (Advanced Life Support Group, 2011).

Care should be taken not to press on the soft tissues under the chin as this may obstruct the airway. Blind finger sweeps are also not recommended (Resuscitation Council (UK), 2011). Although cervical spine injuries are rare in infants and children (American Heart Association, 2000), the jaw thrust rather than head tilt–chin lift is recommended if there is a history of trauma (Advanced Life Support Group, 2011).

Principles of mouth to mouth ventilation

Mouth to mouth ventilation is a quick, effective way to provide adequate oxygenation and ventilation to a casualty who is not breathing. However, particular attention must be paid to the correct technique. The most common cause of failure to ventilate is improper positioning of the head and chin.

Procedure for mouth and nose ventilation (infant)

1. Position the infant in a supine position (preferably on a table or similar flat surface).
2. Place the infant's head in a neutral position and maintain the head tilt and chin lift.
3. If trained to do so, apply a face shield barrier device (if immediately available).
4. Take a deep breath in.

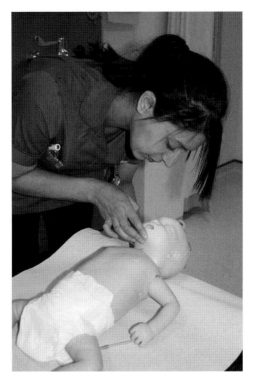

Fig. 4.6 Mouth to mouth and nose ventilation in an infant.

5. Bend forwards from the hips, leaning down towards the infant's nose and mouth (Fig. 4.6).
6. Place your lips around the infant's lips and nose, and ensure an airtight seal.
7. Breathe out steadily into the infant's mouth and nose over 1–1.5 seconds and observe for chest rise (Resuscitation Council (UK), 2011). The correct breath volume is one that causes the chest to rise without causing excessive gastric distension (Berg *et al.*, 1998).
8. While still maintaining head tilt and chin lift, remove your mouth and watch for chest fall as the air comes out.
9. Take another breath in (pausing to take a breath will maximise the oxygen content and minimise the carbon dioxide content in the delivered breaths; Tendrup *et al.*, 1989) and repeat steps 5–9.

If the rescuer has a small mouth, it may not be possible to cover both the infant's nose and mouth (Dembofsky *et al.*, 1999). In this situation, mouth to nose ventilation may be adequate (Tonkin *et al.*, 1995).

Procedure for mouth to mouth ventilation (child)

1. Position the child in a supine position (for a smaller child, preferably on a table or similar).
2. Kneel in a comfortable position with your knees shoulder width apart, at the side of the child at the level of his or her nose and mouth.
3. Rest back to sit on your heels in the low kneeling position.
4. Place the child's head in a 'sniffing the morning air' position and maintain the head tilt and chin lift.
5. If trained to do so, apply a face shield barrier device.
6. Pinch the soft part of the child's nose.
7. Take a deep breath in.
8. Bend forwards from the hips, leaning down towards the child's nose and mouth (Fig. 4.7).
9. Place your lips around the child's lips and ensure an airtight seal.
10. Breathe out steadily into the child's mouth over 1–1.5 seconds and observe for chest rise (Resuscitation Council (UK), 2011). The correct breath volume is one that causes the chest to rise without causing excessive gastric distension (Berg *et al.*, 1998).
11. While still maintaining head tilt and chin lift, remove your mouth and watch for chest fall as the air comes out.
12. Take another breath (as pausing to take a breath will maximise the oxygen content and minimise the carbon dioxide content in the delivered breaths; Tendrup *et al.*, 1989) and repeat steps 8–11.

Ineffective delivery of breaths

If it is difficult to deliver effective breaths (Biarent *et al.*, 2010; Resuscitation Council (UK), 2011):

- Ensure an adequate head tilt and chin lift; the jaw thrust (see Chapter 5) may help.
- Reposition the airway (a slight readjustment may be all that is required).

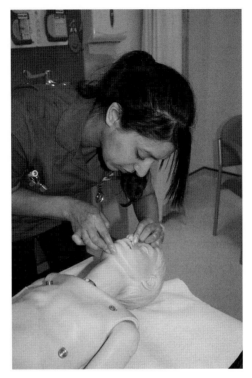

Fig. 4.7 Mouth to mouth ventilation in a child.

- Recheck the child's mouth, and remove any obstruction.
- Ensure the casualty's nose is pinched during ventilation.
- Allow up to five attempts to achieve effective breaths. If the procedure proves unsuccessful, proceed to chest compressions.

Complications of gastric inflation

Gastric inflation is commonly associated with mouth to mouth ventilation, particularly if the rescue breaths are performed rapidly (Melker, 1985). It occurs when the pressure in the oesophagus exceeds the opening pressure of the lower oesophageal sphincter pressure, resulting in the sphincter's opening. During CPR, the oesophageal sphincter relaxes, thus increasing the likelihood of gastric inflation.

The complications of gastric inflation (Berg *et al.*, 1998) include:

- Regurgitation
- Aspiration
- Pneumonia
- Diaphragm elevation, restricted lung movements and reduced lung compliance.

Gastric inflation can be minimised if the rescue breaths are delivered slowly (over 1–1.5 seconds). Correctly applied cricoid pressure (see Chapter 5) may also help.

Principles of performing chest compressions

Push hard and fast. (Biarent *et al.*, 2010)

Mechanisms of blood flow during chest compression

Chest compressions create blood flow by increasing intrathoracic pressure or directly compressing the heart (Maier *et al.*, 1984). Even if chest compressions are being performed correctly, cardiac output is still only about 30% of normal, with systolic blood pressures of between 60 and 80 mmHg being achieved (Paradis *et al.*, 1989). During chest compressions, the blood flow can be maximised by positioning the patient horizontally, using the recommended chest compression force, duration, rate and ratio.

Compression:ventilation ratios

Practitioners with a duty to respond should learn and use a 15:2 compression:ventilation (CV) ratio because this has been validated in animal and manikin studies (Berg *et al.*, 1999; Babbs & Kern, 2002; Dorph *et al.*, 2002; Turner *et al.*, 2002; Babbs & Nadkarni, 2004). However, a lone practitioner may wish to consider a 30:2 CV ratio, particularly if an adequate number of compressions cannot be achieved because of difficulty in the transition between ventilation and compression (Biarent *et al.*, 2010).

Those who are unable or unwilling to provide mouth to mouth ventilation should be encouraged to perform at least compression-only CPR (Resuscitation Council (UK), 2011).

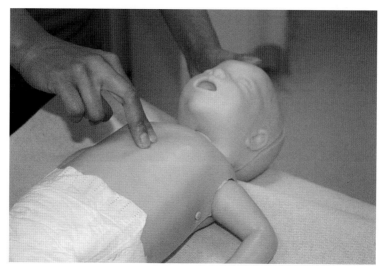

Fig. 4.8 Chest compressions in an infant: two-finger technique.

Chest compressions in an infant

To perform chest compressions in an infant, the two-finger technique (Fig. 4.8) is recommended for a single rescuer, and the two-thumb encircling the rib cage technique (Fig. 4.9) for two or more rescuers (David, 1988; Menegazzi *et al.*, 1993; Houri *et al.*, 1997; Dorfsman *et al.*, 2000; Whitelaw *et al.*, 2000).

The two-thumb technique is usually just used in the in-hospital resuscitation situation (Resuscitation Council (UK), 2011). Two thumbs are placed on the lower half of the sternum (see below), while the rest of the practitioner's hands encircle the infant's chest and back. In very small babies, the thumbs may be positioned one on top of the other.

- *Location* – the lower half of the sternum. Compress the chest one finger's breadth above the xiphisternum (Resuscitation Council (UK), 2011). Compression of the xiphoid process should be avoided as this may injure the liver, stomach or spleen.
- *Depth* – one-third of the anterior–posterior chest diameter (approximately 4 cm in infants).
- *Rate* – at least 100 per minute (but not over 120 per minute).

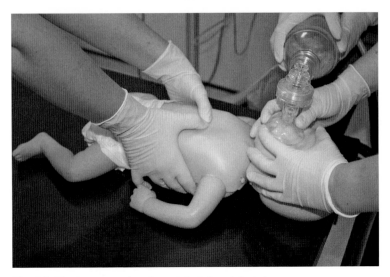

Fig. 4.9 Chest compressions in an infant: thumb technique.

Chest compressions in a child

To perform chest compressions in a child, the use of one hand is recommended (Fig. 4.10); in an older child either the one-hand or two-hands technique (Fig. 4.11) can be used depending on the practitioner's preference (Stevenson *et al.*, 2005). Care should be taken not to apply pressure on the ribs, so ensure that the fingers are clear of the chest. In addition, the arm needs to be straight.

- *Location* – the lower half of the sternum. The heel of one hand is placed on the sternum one finger's breadth above the xiphisternum (Resuscitation Council (UK), 2011). Again, compression of the xiphoid process should be avoided as this may injure the liver, stomach or spleen.
- *Depth* – one third of the anterior–posterior chest diameter (approximately 5 cm in infants).
- *Rate* – at least 100 per minute (but not above 120 per minute).
- *Ratio* – 15 compressions:2 ventilations.

Chest compressions in an older child

In an older child (and in adolescents), the two-handed technique (use in adults) for chest compressions will be required (Resuscitation Council (UK), 2011).

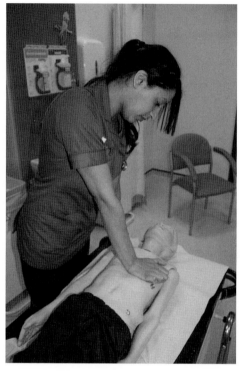

Fig. 4.10 Chest compressions in a child: one-hand technique.

Duration of chest compressions

Cerebral and coronary perfusion is optimum when 50% of the cycle is devoted to the chest compression phase and 50% to the chest relaxation phase (Jevon, 2009). Following chest compression, subsequent complete release is paramount (Biarent *et al.*, 2010).

Rate of chest compression

A chest compression rate of at least 100 per minute (but not over 120 per minute) is required to achieve optimum blood flow during CPR. The rate refers to the speed of compressions rather than the actual number delivered per minute (Resuscitation Council (UK), 2011). Once the child has been intubated and chest compressions and ventilations are asynchronous, the number of

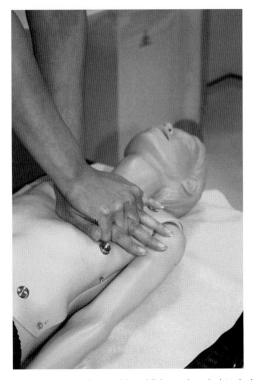

Fig. 4.11 Chest compressions in an older child: two-handed technique.

compressions delivered will then be at least 100, but not over 120, per minute.

The recovery position

Indications

The recovery position is designed to help maintain a patent airway and reduce the risk of airway obstruction and aspiration (American Heart Association, 2005). It is recommended in an unconscious child who is breathing normally and has an effective circulation (American Heart Association, 2005). The recovery position is also recommended in many other situations where the patient's level of consciousness is compromised, e.g. following a major seizure (Bingham, 2004; Hayes, 2004) and during a hypogly-caemic coma (Diebel, 1999).

Key principles

Although a number of recovery positions are currently advocated, no single one can be endorsed. However, the position adopted should:

- Be stable
- Maintain a patent airway
- Maintain a stable cervical spine
- Avoid application of pressure to the chest that restricts breathing
- Minimise the risk of aspiration
- Limit pressure on bony prominences and peripheral nerves
- Enable visualisation of the child's breathing and colour
- Allow access to the child for interventions
- Be easy and safe to achieve (including repositioning if required)

Spinal injury

If the child has a known or suspected spinal injury, he or she should only be moved if an open airway cannot otherwise be maintained. If it is necessary to move the child, e.g. because of a compromised airway, the child should ideally be carefully log-rolled, with the head and neck kept as still as possible and in alignment. Extension of the lower arm above the head together with bending both legs, while rolling the head onto the arm, may be feasible (American Heart Association, 2005).

Right or left lateral

Historically, the left lateral position has been advocated for the recovery position (Eastwick-Field, 1996). However, there appears to be no advantages in terms of cardiac autonomic tone to be gained by placing a person in the recovery position on one side compared with the other (Ryan *et al.*, 2003). Although either side can be used, the environment can in practical terms dictate which side is used; for example, if the child has collapsed next to a wall, he or she will have to be rolled away from it.

A suggested technique

The adult recovery position is suitable for use in children (Biarent *et al.*, 2010). The procedure for this (Resuscitation Council (UK), 2011) is as follows:

1. Check the environment and decide which side is best to roll the child onto. If necessary, remove any obstacles.
2. If necessary, remove the child's spectacles and place them in a safe place.
3. Loosen any clothing around the child's neck.
4. Kneel beside the child. To minimise the risk of self-injury, adopt a stable base with the knees shoulder width apart, avoid twisting your back and keep your spine in a neutral position (Resuscitation Council (UK), 2001).
5. Ensure that both the child's legs are straight.
6. Position the arm nearest to the practitioner perpendicular to the child's body, with the elbow bent and the hand palm uppermost.
7. Grasp the far arm and bring it across the child's chest. Hold the back of the hand against the child's cheek.
8. Using the free hand, grasp the far leg just above the knee and pull it up, taking care to keep the child's foot on the ground
9. While holding the child's hand against his or her cheek, pull on the far leg to roll the child towards you onto his or her side.
10. Adjust the child's upper leg, ensuring that both the hip and the knee are bent at right angles.
11. Tilt the child's head back to ensure that the airway remains open.
12. If necessary, adjust the hand under the child's cheek to maintain the head tilt.
13. Monitor the child's vital signs.

In infants, the support of a small pillow or a rolled-up blanket placed behind the back may be required to help ensure that the position is stable (Resuscitation Council (UK), 2005).

Complications

Even if the child is in the recovery position, the airway, breathing and circulation can still become compromised. Closely monitor the patient's vitals signs, particularly the breathing (Handley *et al.*, 2005).

It has been reported that, when the lower arm is placed in front, compression of vessels and nerves in the dependent limb can occur (Fulstow & Smith, 1993; Turner *et al.*, 1997). Therefore monitor for signs of impaired blood flow in the lowermost arm (Rathgeber *et al.*, 1996) and ensure that the duration over which pressure is exerted on this arm is kept to a minimum (Resuscitation Council (UK), 2011). If the patient needs to remain in the recovery position for longer than 30 minutes, turn him or her to the opposite side to relieve the pressure on the forearm (Biarent *et al.*, 2010).

Management of foreign body airway obstruction

Foreign body airway obstruction (FBAO; choking) is a life-threatening emergency. Case reports have demonstrated the effectiveness of back blows, abdominal thrusts and chest thrusts for the treatment of FBAO (ILCOR, 2005), successful treatment often requiring more than one particular intervention.

Incidence

FBAO is an uncommon, yet potentially treatable, cause of accidental death (Fingerhut *et al.*, 1998). Each year in the UK, approximately 16000 adults and children receive treatment in A&E departments for FBAO (Handley *et al.*, 2005); less than 1% of these incidents are fatal (Industry DoTa, 1999a). In adults, the most common cause of FBAO is food, e.g. meat, poultry and fish (Industry DoTa, 1999a); in children, half of the cases are caused by food (usually sweets), and half are caused by such items as toys, coins, etc. (Industry DoTa, 1999b).

Complete obstruction of the airway by a foreign body is a life-threatening emergency and is often characterised by a sudden inability to talk, maximal respiratory effort, development of cyanosis and clutching of the neck.

In partial airway obstruction, the child will be distressed, may cough and may have a wheeze. In complete airway obstruction, the child will be unable to speak, breathe or cough, and will eventually become unconscious.

Recognition of foreign body airway obstruction

Biarent *et al.* (2010) have listed the signs of FBAO:

- General signs of FBAO
- A witnessed episode
- Coughing/choking
- Sudden onset
- A recent history of playing with or eating small objects

Treatment of choking

The Resuscitation Council (UK) (2011) algorithm for the treatment of choking in infants and children is detailed in Fig. 4.12. The treatment depends on whether the child has an effective or an ineffective cough (Biarent *et al.*, 2010):

- *Effective cough* – the child may be crying or able to provide a verbal response to questions, have a loud cough, have had the ability to breathe before coughing and be fully responsive.
- *Ineffective cough* – there may be inability to vocalise, inability to breathe, a quiet or silent cough, cyanosis or a decreasing level of consciousness.

Treatment of a choking infant

If the infant is choking but able to breathe, encourage him or her to cough. If the infant is choking and is unable to breathe, or shows signs of becoming weak, or stops breathing or coughing, call for help and do the following:

1. Remove any obvious foreign body from the mouth, but do not perform blind finger sweeps as these may further impact the foreign body and may cause pharyngeal trauma (Resuscitation Council (UK), 2011).
2. Position the infant in a prone position resting on your forearm, with the head lower than the chest and the airway open. Ensure the head is well supported.
3. Deliver up to five back blows (Fig. 4.13) between the scapulae using the heel of the hand. If the back blows fail to dislodge the foreign body, proceed to chest thrusts.
4. Turn the infant into a supine position, with the head lower than the chest and the airway open.
5. Deliver up to five chest thrusts to the lower half of the sternum (similar to chest compressions, but more vigorous, sharper and slower) (Fig. 4.14).
6. Recheck the mouth and carefully remove any visible foreign body.
7. If the airway remains obstructed, repeat steps 2–6 as appropriate.

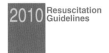

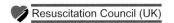

Adult Basic Life Support

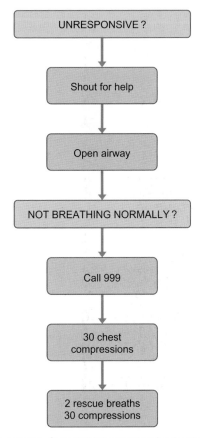

Fig. 4.12 Resuscitation Council (UK) algorithm for the treatment of paediatric foreign body airway obstruction. Reproduced with kind permission of the Resuscitation Council (UK).

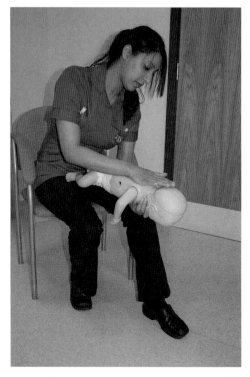

Fig. 4.13 Treatment of foreign body airway obstruction in an infant:
back blows.

If the infant becomes unconscious, call for help and inspect the
airway. If a foreign body is seen, attempt to remove it with a
single finger sweep, open the airway (head tilt and chin lift) and
attempt five ventilations. If chest rise is not seen, slight repositioning of the head is recommended before continuing with ventilations. Chest compressions will need to be started if there is no
response to the ventilation and the infant remains unconscious.
Chest compressions could generate sufficient pressure to remove
the foreign body (Langelle *et al.*, 2000).

Abdominal thrusts are not recommended in infants (Resuscitation Council (UK), 2011).

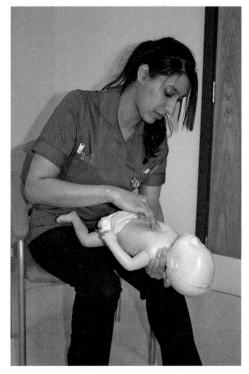

Fig. 4.14 Treatment of foreign body airway obstruction in an infant: chest thrusts.

Treatment of a choking child

If the child is choking but able to breathe, encourage him to cough. If the child is choking and is unable to breathe, or shows signs of becoming weak, or stops breathing or coughing, call for help and do the following:

1. Remove any obvious foreign body from the mouth, but do not perform blind finger sweeps as these may further impact the foreign body and may cause pharyngeal trauma (Resuscitation Council (UK), 2011).
2. Position the child head down.
3. Deliver up to five back blows (Fig. 4.15) between the scapulae using the heel of the hand. If the back blows fail to dislodge the foreign body, proceed to abdominal thrusts.

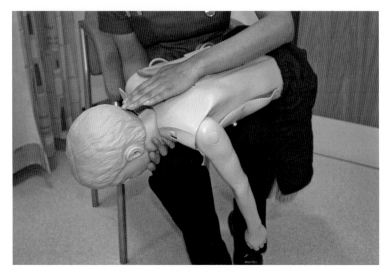

Fig. 4.15 Treatment of foreign body airway obstruction in a child: back blows.

4. Stand or kneel behind the child.
5. Position your arms directly underneath the child's axillae and encircle the torso.
6. Bend the child forward.
7. Place the thumb side of one fist against the child's abdomen, in the midline just above the umbilicus but well below the xiphoid process.
8. Grasp the fist with the other hand.
9. Exert up to five quick inward and upward thrusts. Avoid touching the xiphoid process and lower margins of the rib cage because any force applied to these structures could damage the internal organs. Recheck the mouth and carefully remove any visible foreign body.
10. If the airway remains obstructed, repeat steps 2–6 as appropriate.

If the child becomes unconscious, call for help and inspect the airway. If a foreign body is seen, attempt to remove it with a single finger sweep, open the airway (head tilt and chin lift) and attempt five ventilations. If chest rise is not seen, slight repositioning of the head is recommended before continuing with ventilations. Chest compressions will need to be started if there is no response to the ventilations and the child remains unconscious. Chest compressions could generate sufficient pressure to remove the foreign body (Langelle *et al.*, 2000).

Principles of safer handling during CPR

The Resuscitation Council (UK), in its publication *Guidance for Safer Handling During Resuscitation in Hospitals* (2001), has issued guidelines concerning safer handling during CPR. Although these are mainly aimed at the resuscitation of adults, some are applicable to paediatric resuscitation. A brief overview of these guidelines will now be provided.

- *Environmental hazards* – remove any hazards. Ensure that the bed (resuscitaire) brakes are on, and lower cotsides if they are up.
- *Ventilation and intubation* – move the bed away from the wall and remove the backrest to allow access. Stand at the top of the bed facing the child with your feet in a walk/stand position and avoid prolonged static postures.
- *Chest compressions* – ensure the bed is at a height that places the child between the knee and mid-thigh of the practitioner performing the chest compressions; stand at the side of the bed with the feet shoulder width apart and position the shoulders directly over the child's sternum. Keeping the arms straight, compress the chest, ensuring that the force for compression results from flexing the hips; chest compressions can also be performed by kneeling with both knees on the bed.
- *CPR on a fixed-height bed, couch or trolley* – if necessary, stand on steps or a firm stool with a non-slip surface and that is wide enough to permit your feet to be shoulder width apart; do not kneel on a couch or trolley.

Summary

The initial assessment and sequence of actions in BLS in infants and children has been discussed. The principles of basic airway management, ventilation and chest compressions have been described, and the management of FBAO has been outlined. As respiratory failure is the most common cause of cardiac arrest in childhood, particular attention to securing the airway and providing adequate ventilation is paramount.

References

Abernethy, J.L., Allan, P.L. & Drummond, G.B. (1990) Ultrasound assessment of the position of the tongue during induction of anaesthesia. *British Journal of Anaesthesia*, **65**, 744–748.

Advanced Life Support Group (2011) *Advanced Paediatric Life Support*, 5th edn. Wiley, Oxford.

American Heart Association (2005) 2005 American Heart Association Guidelines for Cardiopulmonary Resuscitation and Emergency Cardiovascular Care. *Circulation*, **112**, 24 (Suppl).

Babbs, C. & Kern, K. (2002) Optimum compression to ventilation ratios in CPR under realistic, practical conditions: a physiological and mathematical analysis. *Resuscitation*, **54**, 147–157.

Babbs, C. & Nadkarni, V. (2004) Optimizing chest compression to rescue ventilation ratios during one-rescuer CPR by professionals and lay persons: children are not just little adults. *Resuscitation*, **61**, 173–181.

Berg, M., Idris, A. & Berg, R. (1998) Severe ventilatory compromise due to gastric distension during pediatric cardiopulmonary resuscitation. *Resuscitation*, **36**, 71–73.

Berg, R., Hilwig, R., Kern, K., *et al.* (1999) Simulated mouth-to-mouth ventilation and chest compressions (bystander cardiopulmonary resuscitation) improves outcome in a swine model of prehospital pediatric asphyxial cardiac arrest. *Critical Care Medicine*, **27**, 1893–1899.

Biarent, D., Bingham, R. & Christoph, E., *et al.* (2010) European Resuscitation Council Guidelines for Resuscitation Section 6. Paediatric life support (2010). *Resuscitation*, **81**, 1364–1388.

Bingham, E. (2004) Epilepsy: diagnosis and support for people with epilepsy. *Practice Nursing*, **15**(2), 64–70.

David, R. (1988) Closed chest cardiac massage in the newborn infant. *Pediatrics*, **81**, 552–554.

Dembofsky, C.A., Gibson, E., Nadkarni, V., *et al.* (1999) Assessment of infant cardiopulmonary resuscitation rescue breathing technique: relationship of infant and caregiver facial measurements. *Pediatrics*, **103**, E17.

Diebel, G. (1999) The management of hypoglycaemia in type1 and type 2 diabetes. *British Journal of Community Nursing*, **4**(9), 454–460.

Dorfsman, M., Menegazzi, J., Wadas, R. & Auble, T. (2000) Two-thumb vs two-finger chest compression in an infant model of prolonged cardiopulmonary resuscitation. *Academy of Emergency Medicine*, **7**, 1077–1082.

Dorph, E., Wik, L. & Steen, P. (2002) Effectiveness of ventilation-compression ratios 1:5 and 2:15 in simulated single rescuer paediatric resuscitation. *Resuscitation*, **54**, 259–264.

Eastwick-Field, P. (1996) Resuscitation: basic life support. *Nursing Standard*, **10**, 49–56.

Fingerhut, L., Cox, C. & Warner, M. (1998) International comparative analysis of injury mortality. Findings from the ICE on injury statistics. International collaborative effort on injury statistics. *Advance Data*, **12**, 1–20.

Friesen, R.M., Duncan, P. & Tweed, W. (1982) Appraisal of pediatric cardiopulmonary resuscitation. *Canadian Medical Association Journal*, **126**, 1055–1058.

Fulstow, R. & Smith, G. (1993) The new recovery position, a cautionary tale. *Resuscitation*, **26**, 89–91.

Handley, A., Koster, R. & Monsieurs, K. *et al.* (2005) European Resuscitation Council Guidelines for Resuscitation 2005: Section 2. Adult basic life support and use of automated external defibrillators. *Resuscitation*, **67**, S1, S7–S23.

Hayes, C. (2004) Clinical skills: practical guide for managing adults with epilepsy. *British Journal of Nursing*, **13**, 380–387.

Hazinski, M.F. (1995) Is paediatric resuscitation unique? Relative merits of early CPR and ventilation versus early defibrillation for young victims of cardiac arrest. *Annals of Emergency Medicine*, **25**, 540–543.

Houri, P., Frank, L., Menegazzi, J. & Taylor, R. (1997) A randomized, controlled trial of two-thumb vs two-finger chest compression in a swine infant model of cardiac arrest. *Prehospital Emergency Care*, **1**, 65–67.

Hugdel, D.W. & Hendricks, C. (1988) Palate and hypopharynx: sites of inspiratory narrowing of the upper airway during sleep. *American Review of Respiratory Disease*, **138**, 1542–1547.

ILCOR (2005) Part 2: Adult basic life support. 2005 International Consensus on Cardiopulmonary Resuscitation and Emergency Cardiovascular Care Science with Treatment Recommendations. *Resuscitation*, **67**, 187–200.

Industry DoTa (1999a) *Choking in Home and Leisure Accident Report*. Department of Trade and Industry, London.

Industry DoTa (1999b) *Choking Risks for Children*. Department of Trade and Industry, London.

Jevon P (2009) *Advanced Cardiac Life Support*, 2nd edn. Wiley Blackwell, Oxford.

Kitamura, T., Iwami, T., Kawamura, T., *et al.* (2010) Conventional and chest-compression only cardiopulmonary resuscitation by bystanders for children who have out-of- hospital cardiac arrests: a prospective, nationwide, population-based cohort. *Lancet*, **375**, 1347–1354.

Langelle, A., Sunde, K., Wik, L. & Steen, P. (2000) Airway pressure with chest compressions versus Heimlich manoeuvre in recently dead adults with complete airway obstruction. *Resuscitation*, **44**, 105–108.

Maier, M.D., Tyson, G.S., Jr., Olsen, C.O., *et al.* (1984) The physiology of external cardiac massage: high impulse cardiopulmonary resuscitation Circulation; **70**, 86–101

Melker, R.J. & Banner, M.J. (1985) Ventilation during CPR: two-rescuer standards reappraised. *Annals of Emergency Medicine*, **14**, 397–402.

Menegazzi, J., Auble, T., Nicklas, K. *et al.* (1993) Two-thumb versus two-finger chest compression during CRP in a swine infant model of cardiac arrest. *Annals of Emergency Medicine*, **22**, 240–243.

Noc, M., Weil, M., Sus, S., *et al* (1994) Spontaneous gasping during cardiopulmonary resuscitation without mechanical ventilation. *American Journal of Respiratory and Critical Care Medicine*, **150**, 861–864.

Paradis, N., Martin, G.B., Goetting, M.G., *et al.* (1989) Simultaneous aortic, jugular bulb, and right atrial pressures during cardiopulmonary resuscitation in humans. Insights into mechanisms. *Circulation*, **80**, 361–368.

Poets, C., Meny, R., Chobanian, M. & Bonofiglo, R. (1999) Gasping and other cardiorespiratory patterns during sudden infant deaths. *Pediatric Research*, **45**, 350–354.

Rathgeber, J., Panzer, W., Gunther, U., *et al.* (1996) Influence of different types of recovery positions on perfusion indices of the forearm. *Resuscitation*, **32**, 13–17.

Resuscitation Council (UK) (2001) *Guidance for Safer Handling During Resuscitation in Hospitals*. Resuscitation Council (UK), London.

Resuscitation Council (UK) (2005) *Guidelines 2005*. Resuscitation Council (UK), London.

Resuscitation Council (UK) (2011) *Paediatric Immediate Life Support*, 2nd edn. Resuscitation Council (UK), London.

Roth, B., Magnusson, J., Joahansson, I., *et al* (1998) Jaw lift: a simple and effective method to open the airway in children. *Resuscitation*, **39**, 171–174.

Ruben, H.M., Elam, J.O. & Ruben, A.M. (1961) Investigation of upper airway problems in resuscitation. Studies of pharyngeal X-rays and performance by lay men. *Anesthesiology*, **22**, 271–279.

Ruppert, M., Reith, M., Widdman, J., *et al.* (1999) Checking for breathing: evaluation of the diagnostic capability of emergency medical services personnel, physicians, medical students and medical laypersons. *Annals of Emergency Medicine*, **34**, 720–729.

Ryan, A., Larsen, P. & Galletly, D. (2003) Comparison of heart rate variability in supine, and left and right lateral positions. *Anaesthesia*, **58**, 432–436.

Safranek, D., Eisenberg, M. & Larsen, M. (1992) The epidemiology of cardiac arrest in young adults. *Annals of Emergency Medicine*, **21**, 1102–1106.

Sarti, A., Savron, F., Casotto, V. & Cuttini, M. (2005) Heartbeat assessment in infants: a comparison of four clinical methods. *Pediatric Critical Care Medicine*, **6**, 212–215.

Sarti, A., Savron, F., Ronfani, L., *et al.* (2006) Comparison of three sites to check the pulse and count heart rate in hypotensive infants. *Paediatric Anaesthesia*, **16**, 394–398.

Stevenson, A., McGowan, J., Evans, A. & Graham, C. (2005) CPR for children: one hand or two? *Resuscitation*, **64**, 205–208.

Tendrup, T., Kanter, R. & Cherry, R. (1989) A comparison of infant ventilation methods performed by pre-hospital personnel. *Annals of Emergency Medicine*, **18**, 607–611.

Tibballs, J. & Weeranatna, C. (2010) The influence of time on the accuracy of healthcare personnel to diagnose paediatric cardiac arrest by pulse palpation. *Resuscitation*, **81**, 671–675.

Tibballs, J., Carter, B., Kiraly, N., *et al.* (2010) External and internal biphasic direct current shock doses for pediatric ventricular fibrillation and pulseless ventricular tachycardia. *Pediatric Critical Care Medicine*, **12**, 14–20.

Tonkin, S., Davis, S. & Gunn, T. (1995) Nasal route for infant resuscitation by mothers. *Lancet*, **345**, 1353–1354.

Turner, I., Turner, S. & Armstrong, V. (2002) Does the compression to ventilation ratio affect the quality of CPR: a simulation study. *Resuscitation*, **52**, 55–62.

Turner, S., Turner, I., Chapman, D., *et al.* (1997) A comparative study of the 1992 and 1997 recovery positions for use in the UK. *Resuscitation*, **39**, 153–160.

Whitelaw, C.C., Slywka, B. & Goldsmith, L. (2000) Comparison of a two-finger versus two thumb method for chest compressions by healthcare providers in an infant mechanical model. *Resuscitation*, **43**, 213–216.

Chapter 5

Airway Management and Ventilation

Introduction

The priorities and sequence of paediatric basic life support (BLS) follow the principle that early effective oxygenation and ventilation must be established as quickly as possible (Resuscitation Council (UK), 2011a). Indeed, survival from cardiopulmonary arrest is mainly dependent upon the immediate provision of effective rescue ventilations (Friesen *et al.*, 1982). Effective airway management and ventilation during cardiopulmonary resuscitation is therefore paramount.

The aim of this chapter is to understand the principles of airway management and ventilation.

Learning objectives

At the end of this chapter, the reader will be able to:

- Discuss the relevant anatomy and physiology
- List the causes of airway obstruction
- Outline the recognition of airway obstruction
- Describe simple techniques to open and clear the airway
- Discuss the procedure for the application of cricoid pressure
- Discuss the use of oropharyngeal and nasopharyngeal airways
- Outline the role of the laryngeal mask airway
- Describe the procedure for tracheal intubation
- Describe two methods of ventilation

Paediatric Advanced Life Support: A Practical Guide for Nurses, Second Edition.
Phil Jevon.
© 2012 Phil Jevon. Published 2012 by Blackwell Publishing Ltd.

Relevant anatomy and physiology

Anatomical changes

As the child's weight increases with age, the size, shape and proportions of the various organs also change. Particular anatomical changes are relevant to emergency care.

Airway

- *A large head and short neck* – these can cause neck flexion and narrowing of the airway.
- *A small face and mandible* – these make airway intervention more difficult.
- *Teeth and orthodontic appliances* – as these may be loose.
- *A relatively large tongue* – this can obstruct the airway in an unconscious child and can make laryngoscopy difficult.
- *The floor of the mouth is easily compressed* – care should be taken when positioning the fingers while performing airway manoeuvres.
- *Infants under 6 months old are nasal breathers* – their narrow nasal passages can easily become obstructed by mucous secretions (as upper respiratory tract infections are common in infants less than 6 months), which may lead to the airway becoming compromised.
- *3–8-year-olds may have adenotonsillar hypertrophy* – this can cause obstruction and may hinder the insertion of a pharyngeal, gastric or tracheal tube via the nasal route.
- *The epiglottis in all young children is horseshoe-shaped and projects posteriorly at 45 degrees* – making tracheal intubation is more difficult.
- *The larynx is positioned higher and more anteriorly* – tracheal intubation in infants is usually easier with a straight-blade laryngoscope.
- *The cricoid cartilage (compared with the larynx in adults) is the narrowest part of the upper airway* – blind finger sweeps could inadvertently push a foreign body down to this level, making removal very difficult. The cricoid cartilage is also particularly susceptible to oedema.
- *A short and soft trachea* – overextension or flexion of the neck could kink the trachea. In addition, a tracheal tube can more easily become displaced.

- *High compliance of the airway* – this makes it very susceptible to dynamic collapse when it is obstructed (Wittenborg *et al.*, 1967).

Breathing

- *Relatively narrow upper and lower airways* – these are more easily obstructed, and because resistance to flow of air is inversely proportional to the fourth power of the airway radius (so that halving the radius increases the resistance 16-fold), even a small reduction in airway size can lead to a significant increase in airflow resistance and work of breathing. This is particularly true if the airflow is turbulent, e.g. during crying (Cote & Todres, 1990) – hence why children with airway obstruction should be kept as calm and quiet as possible.
- *Infants rely mainly on the diaphragm for breathing* – their muscles are more prone to fatigue, which could lead to respiratory failure.
- *The ribs in infants are positioned horizontally* – they contribute less to chest expansion during breathing.
- *Ribs and intercostal cartilage are very compliant* – they may fail to support breathing (Mansell *et al.*, 1972).

Physiological changes

- *High oxygen demand due to high metabolic rate* – per kilogram weight, oxygen consumption in infants is twice of that in adults (Cross *et al.*, 1957).

(Source: Advanced Life Support Group, 2011; Resuscitation Council (UK), 2011a)

Causes of airway obstruction

Causes of airway obstruction include:

- *Displaced tongue* – causes include unconsciousness, cardiac arrest and trauma
- *Fluid* – e.g. vomit, secretions and blood
- *Foreign body*

- *Laryngeal oedema* – causes include anaphylaxis and infection
- *Bronchospasm* – causes include asthma, foreign body and anaphylaxis
- *Trauma*
- *Pulmonary oedema* – causes include cardiac failure, anaphylaxis and near-drowning

Recognition of airway obstruction

Whatever the cause of airway obstruction, prompt recognition and effective management are essential. Recognition is best achieved by following the familiar look, listen and feel approach (Resuscitation Council (UK), 2011a):

- *Look* for movements of the chest and abdomen
- *Listen* at the mouth and nose for airflow
- *Feel* at the mouth and nose for airflow.

Airway obstruction can be partial or complete, and can occur at any level from the nose and mouth down to the trachea.

Partial airway obstruction

Partial airway obstruction is usually characterised by noisy breathing:

- *Gurgling* – the presence of fluid, e.g. secretions in the main airways
- *Snoring* – partial occlusion of the pharynx by the tongue
- *Crowing* – laryngeal spasm
- *Inspiratory stridor* – upper airway obstruction (at or above the level of the larynx), e.g. foreign body or croup
- *Expiratory wheeze* – lower airway obstruction, e.g. asthma

Complete airway obstruction

Complete airway obstruction in a child who is making respiratory efforts is characterised by paradoxical chest and abdominal movements ('see-saw' breathing) – on trying to breathe in, the chest is drawn inwards and the abdomen expands, the opposite happening when the child is trying to breathe out.

Simple techniques to open and clear the airway

The airway in an unconscious child can easily become obstructed by a combination of flexion of the neck, relaxation of the jaw, displacement of the tongue against the posterior wall of the pharynx and collapse of the hypopharynx (Hugdel & Hendricks, 1988; Abernethy *et al.*, 1990). In some cases, just opening the airway may revive the child.

Head tilt–chin lift

The airway can be opened by tilting the head and lifting the chin. This will help to open the airway and bring the tongue forward from the posterior wall of the pharynx (the tongue being most common cause of airway obstruction in an unconscious child; Ruben *et al.*, 1961). The neutral position in an infant (Fig. 5.1) and the 'sniffing the morning air' position in a child (Fig. 5.2) are recommended (Advanced Life Support Group, 2011). Care should be

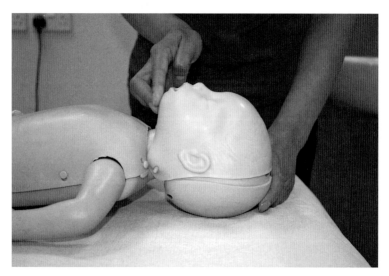

Fig. 5.1 Opening the airway: head tilt–chin lift (neutral position in an infant).

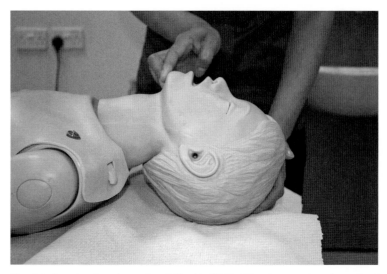

Fig. 5.2 Opening the airway: head tilt–chin lift ('sniffing the morning air position' in a child).

taken not to press on the soft tissues under the chin as this may obstruct the airway. Blind finger sweeps are not recommended.

Jaw thrust

The jaw thrust is considered to be4 the most effective method of opening the airway in a child (Resuscitation Council (UK), 2011a). It is definitely advocated if there is a suspected or confirmed cervical spine injury. To perform a jaw thrust (Fig. 5.3):

1. Approach the child from behind.
2. Position two to three fingers under each side of the lower jaw at its angle.
3. Gently rest the thumbs on the child's cheeks.
4. Life the jaw upwards.
5. If required, ensure that a colleague provides manual in-line immobilisation of the head and neck.
6. Check for airway patency.

Suction

When obstruction is caused by vomit, secretions, etc., simple BLS manoeuvres such as placing the child in the lateral position and finger sweeps under direct vision can help to clear the airway.

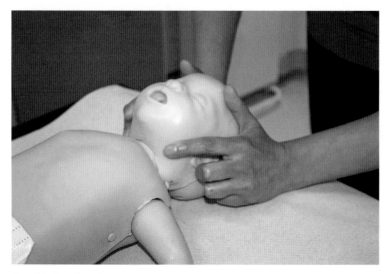

Fig. 5.3 Jaw thrust.

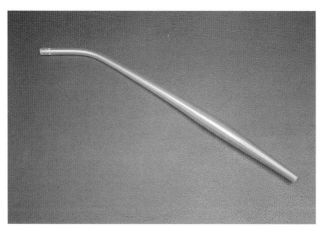

Fig. 5.4 Wide-bore rigid suction catheter.

A wide-bore rigid (Yankauer) catheter (Fig 5.4) can provide rapid suction of large volumes of fluid from the mouth and pharynx. A flexible catheter is particularly useful for suctioning down an oropharyngeal airway, nasopharyngeal airway and tracheal tube. In order to minimise deoxygenation, suction should last no longer than 10 seconds (Jevon, 2009).

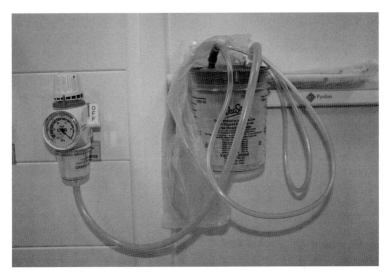

Fig. 5.5 Wall suction device.

A wall suction device is ideal for suction at the bedside (Fig. 5.5). There are also a number portable suction devices currently available that are ideal in some situations, e.g. during patient transfer. Laerdal's Premier Suction Unit is light and durable. It has a variable vacuum regulator that makes it ideal for both paediatric and adult use. It can be operated by either a battery or an external power source. It also has a specially designed filter to protect the collection vessel. A hand-held suction device (Fig. 5.6) is particularly useful in the first aid setting.

Principles of cricoid pressure

Cricoid pressure was first described by Sellick, who advocated its use during the induction of anaesthesia to reduce the incidence of aspiration of gastric contents. Although it can prevent or limit the regurgitation of gastric contents (Salem *et al.*, 1985; Moynihan *et al.*, 1993), it can also distort the airway and make laryngoscopy and tracheal intubation more difficult (Walker *et al.*, 2010).

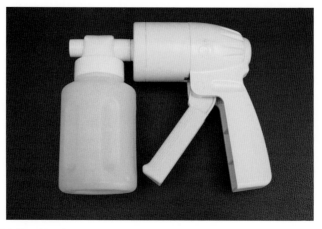

Fig. 5.6 Hand-held suction device.

Technique

1. Palpate a prominent horizontal band below the thyroid cartilage (Adam's apple) and cricothyroid membrane.
2. Apply backward pressure on the cricoid using one fingertip
   in infants, and the thumb and index finger in children. This
   will help to obstruct the lumen of the oesophagus lying posteriorly; if there is a suspected cervical spine injury, counter-
   pressure may be applied to the back of the neck to reduce the
   movement of the cervical spine (Resuscitation Council (UK),
   2011b).
3. Release the cricoid pressure only when a tracheal tube is in
   place to protect the airway (or if the child actively vomits).

Cautions

Cricoid pressure should not be applied during active vomiting
because there is a risk of damage to the oesophagus (Resuscitation Council (UK), 2011b). Too much pressure may compress and
obstruct the trachea and could distort upper airway anatomy
(Hartsilver & Vanner, 2000), making tracheal intubation difficult.
If the application of cricoid pressure impedes ventilation or
hinders tracheal intubation, it should be either modified of
stopped (Biarent *et al.*, 2010).

Oropharyngeal and nasopharyngeal airways

Oropharyngeal (Guedel) and nasopharyngeal airways are useful adjuncts because they can provide an artificial passage to airflow by separating the posterior pharyngeal wall from the tongue. Each will now be discussed in turn.

Oropharyngeal airway

The oropharyngeal airway (Fig. 5.7) can be used when there is obstruction of the upper airway due to the displacement of the tongue backwards, and when the glossopharyngeal and laryngeal reflexes are absent. However, it is usually only used when the head tilt and chin lift have failed to provide a clear airway. It should not be used if the child is not completely unconscious as it may induce vomiting and laryngospasm.

It is important to ensure the correct size is used because:

- If it is too big it may actually block the airway, hinder the use of a face mask and damage the laryngeal structures
- If it is too small, it may block the airway by pushing the tongue back

An appropriately sized airway is one that holds the tongue in the normal anatomical position and follows its natural curvature.

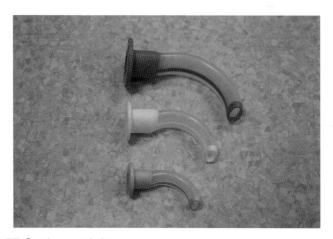

Fig. 5.7 Oropharyngeal airways.

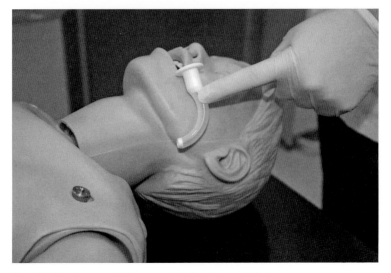

Fig. 5.8 Oropharyngeal airway: estimating the correct size.

The curved body of the oropharyngeal airway is designed to fit over the back of the tongue. The correct size can be estimated by placing the airway against the face and measuring it from the corner of the mouth to the angle of the jaw (Fig. 5.8; Resuscitation Council (UK), 2011a). Various sizes of oropharyngeal airway are currently available.

It is also important to insert the airway correctly in order to avoid unnecessary trauma to the delicate tissues in the mouth and inadvertently block the airway. In older children, the oropharyngeal airway (lubricated if possible) can be inserted into the mouth in the inverted position (as the curved part of the airway will help to depress the tongue and prevent it being pushed posteriorly) and, as it passes over the soft palate, rotated through 180 degrees (Advanced Life Support Group, 2011). Following insertion of the airway, patency of the airway should be checked and the head tilt–chin lift maintained.

In infants, the oropharyngeal airway (lubricated if possible) should be inserted 'right side up' with the tongue depressed out of the way (Advanced Life Support Group, 2011) – if inserted in the inverted position, it may damage the soft palate. Following insertion, the patency of the airway should be checked and the head tilt–chin lift maintained.

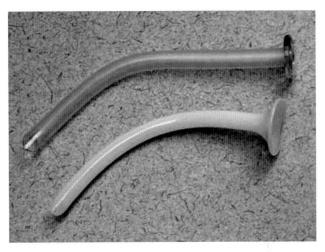

Fig. 5.9 Nasopharyngeal airway.

Nasopharyngeal airway

The nasopharyngeal airway (Fig. 5.9) is preferable if the child is semi-conscious because the risk of gagging, vomiting and laryngospasm is minimal. It is less likely to induce gagging than an oropharyngeal airway, and it can be used in a semi-conscious or conscious child when the airway is at risk of being compromised. It is contraindicated if there is a suspected base of skull fracture (because it may penetrate the cranial fossa) or coagulopathy (Biarent *et al.*, 2010).

Insertion may damage the mucosal lining of the nasal airway, resulting in bleeding. The correct size should be used and prior to insertion, and a safety pin should be securely inserted into the flange to prevent inhalation of the airway.

It is important to estimate the correct length. If it is too short, it will be ineffective, and if it is too long, it may enter the oesophagus, causing distension and hypoventilation, or may stimulate the laryngeal or glossopharyngeal reflexes, causing laryngospasm and vomiting. The correct length of the nasopharyngeal airway is one that equates with the distance from the tip of the nose to the angle of the mandible (Biarent *et al.*, 2010). The correct width is one that does not cause sustained blanching of the alae nasi (American Academy of Pediatrics, 1997).

As paediatric-sized nasopharyngeal airways are not commercially available, a shortened tracheal tube may be used (Advanced

Life Support Group, 2011). Following lubrication, the airway should be gently inserted through the nostril in a posterior direction perpendicular to the plane of the child's face (American Academy of Pediatrics, 1997).

Reassess the airway and check for patency and adequacy of ventilation. Continue to maintain correct alignment of the airway and chin lift as necessary, and monitor the patency of the airway. Suction as necessary.

Role of the laryngeal mask airway

Although bag-mask ventilation remains the recommended first-line method for achieving airway control and ventilation in children, the laryngeal mask airway (LMA; Fig. 5.10) is nevertheless

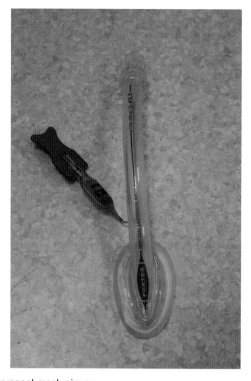

Fig. 5.10 Laryngeal mask airway.

considered an acceptable airway device for providers trained in its use (Rechner *et al.*, 2007; Blevin *et al.*, 2009; Biarent *et al.*, 2010). The LMA is commonly used in adult and paediatric anaesthesia, as well as in adult resuscitation (Advanced Life Support Group, 2011).

The LMA can be particularly helpful when airway obstruction has been caused by a supraglottic airway abnormality or if bag-mask ventilation is not possible (Biarent *et al.*, 2010). Although it can help ventilation, the LMA does not protect the airway against regurgitation and aspiration. In addition, the smaller LMA sizes used in children, although easy to insert, are easy to dislodge (Advanced Life Support Group, 2011). In fact, the LMA is associated with a higher incidence of complications in small children compared with adults (Harnett *et al.*, 2000; Park *et al.*, 2001).

The place of the LMA in the resuscitation of infants and children is still considered to be uncertain, although for those proficient in its use, it may be life-saving in the 'can't intubate, can't ventilate' scenario. It should therefore be available in clinical areas where intubation may be performed (Advanced Life Support Group, 2011).

Principles of tracheal intubation

Tracheal intubation is the most secure and effective method of establishing and maintaining the airway, preventing gastric distension, protecting the lungs against pulmonary aspiration, enabling optimal control of the airway pressure and providing positive end-expiratory pressure (Biarent *et al.*, 2010).

The oral route is preferable during resuscitation because it is quicker, simpler and associated with fewer complications than nasal placement (Biarent *et al.*, 2010). If the child is not unconscious, the judicious use of anaesthetics, sedatives and neuromuscular blocking drugs is essential to improve the chances of success (Wang *et al.*, 2001, 2003; Kaye *et al.*, 2003).

The risk of gastric distension, regurgitation and aspiration of gastric contents, which are not uncommon during BLS, is minimised. However, as the technique can be difficult and sometimes hazardous, regular experience in its use is required.

Indications

Indications for tracheal intubation include:

- Ineffective ventilation
- High peak inspiratory pressures required
- Ineffective bag-valve-mask ventilation
- Prolonged ventilation
- Transfer

Equipment

A suggested list of equipment includes:

- Two laryngoscopes, in working order with appropriate blades
- Tracheal tubes (Fig. 5.11)
- A suction source, including a Yankauer (rigid) suction catheter and a suction catheter of appropriate size to suction down the tracheal tube
- An oxygen source
- Tape to secure the tube
- A stylet
- A ventilation device, e.g. bag-valve-mask
- A stethoscope
- Magill forceps (Fig. 5.12)

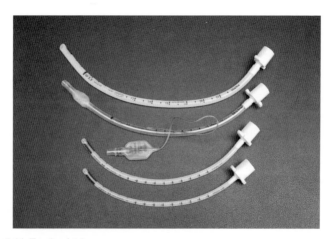

Fig. 5.11 Tracheal tubes.

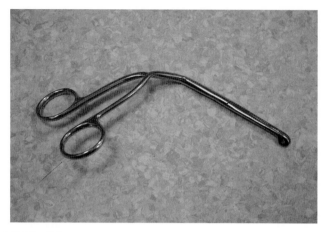

Fig. 5.12 Magill forceps.

Tracheal tubes

Tracheal tubes come in a variety of different designs and sizes. A standard 15 mm adapter is connected to the proximal end, enabling the attachment of a ventilatory device.

The tracheal tube should have distance markers (in centimetres) that provide a point of reference during intubation, and following intubation facilitate the early detection of tube migration.

Tracheal tube sizes

The correctly sized tracheal tube (in millimetres – internal diameter) can be estimated by referring to a paediatric resuscitation chart or a length-based resuscitation tape (remembering that body length is better than body weight at predicting correct the tube size) (Luten *et al.*, 1992). The European Resuscitation Council (Biarent *et al.*, 2010) has provided helpful guidance (Table 5.1). A suggested formula for estimating the correct length (cm) of a tracheal tube is (age/2) + 12 (Advanced Life Support Group, 2011).

Cuffed versus uncuffed tracheal tubes

Although uncuffed tracheal tubes have traditionally been used in children up to 8 years of age, cuffed tubes do offer advantages in certain clinical situations, e.g. poor lung compliance, high

Table 5.1 Recommended cuffed and uncuffed tracheal tube sizes

Age	Uncuffed tracheal tube (internal diameter, mm)	Cuffed tracheal tube (internal diameter, mm)
Neonate premature)	Gestational age in weeks/10	N/A
Newborn (term)	3.5	N/A
<1 year	3.5–4.0	3.0–3.5
Child 1–2 years	4.0–4.5	3.5–4.0
Child > 2 years	Age/4 plus 4	Age/4 plus 3.5

Source: Biarent *et al.* (2010); Resuscitation Council (UK) (2011a).

airway resistance or a large air leak around the glottis (Deakers *et al.*, 1994; Khine *et al.*, 1997; Newth *et al.*, 2004).

Using a correctly sized cuffed tracheal tube is just as safe as using an uncuffed tube for infants (not neonates) and children as long as attention is paid to insertion and cuff inflation pressure (Deakers *et al.*, 1994; Newth *et al.*, 2004). It has also been shown that, when a cuffed tube is used, it is more probable that the correct size will be chosen on the first attempt (Weiss *et al.*, 2009).

As excessive cuff pressure can lead to ischaemic damage to the surrounding
laryngeal tissues and stenosis (Biarent *et al.*, 2010), cuff inflation pressure should be monitored and maintained at less than $25\,cmH_2O$ (Mhanna *et al.*, 2002).

Laryngoscope

The laryngoscope consists of a handle with batteries and a blade with a light source. In modern fibreoptic laryngoscopes, the bulb is situated in the top of the handle rather than in the blade itself – this design feature is preferable because the bulb is secure and protected, and the blade can easily be cleaned after use.

There are two main designs of laryngoscopes blade (Fig. 5.13) for use in children:

- *Straight blade* – this is preferred for infants and small children because it provides better visualisation of the relatively cephalad and anterior glottis (Advanced Life Support Group, 2011). It is designed to pass over the epiglottis and rest at the opening of the glottis. Blade traction (upwards and forwards along the line of the handle) will lift the base of the tongue and the epi-

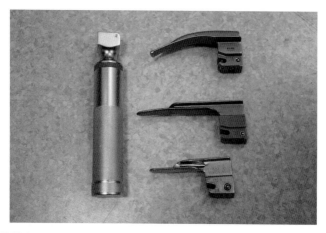

Fig. 5.13 Laryngoscope blades.

glottis anteriorly, and expose the glottis (American Academy of Pediatrics, 2000).
- *Curved blade* – this preferred for older children because the wider base and flange facilitates tongue displacement and improves visualisation of the glottis (Advanced Life Support Group, 2011). The tip of the blade should rest in the vallecula (space between the base of the tongue and the epiglottis). Blade traction (upwards and forwards along the line of the handle) will then displace the base of the tongue anteriorly and expose the glottis (American Academy of Pediatrics, 2000).

The advantage of advancing the blade past the epiglottis is that the latter will then not obscure visualisation of the vocal cords; the advantage of stopping short of the epiglottis is that it will cause less stimulation and will therefore be less likely to cause laryngospasm (Advanced Life Support Group, 2011). Inserting the blade first into the oesophagus and then slowly withdrawing it until the glottis is visualised can cause laryngeal trauma and is not recommended (American Academy of Pediatrics, 1997).

> It is possible to successfully intubate with a blade that is too long, but not with one that is too short (Advanced Life Support Group, 2011).

Procedure for tracheal intubation

1. Ensure that access to the child's head is not restricted. Move the bed away from the wall and remove the backrest if applicable.
2. Assemble the necessary equipment and check to see that it is in good working order.
3. Position yourself at the child's head with your feet in the walk/stand position (Resuscitation Council (UK), 2011a).
4. Correctly position the head – the axes of the mouth, pharynx and trachea should be aligned in order to be able to directly visualise the glottis. For a child aged over 2 years, place the head on a small pillow. This will slightly flex the neck and bring the larynx into optimum alignment for tracheal intubation (Resuscitation Council (UK), 2011a). In infants and children under 2 years of age, the head should be placed on a flat surface – a pillow is not required, although a small rolled-up towel under the shoulders is sometimes used to maintain the position (Resuscitation Council (UK), 2011a). If the neck is overextended, this will lift the glottis out of the line of site, and the trachea may become obstructed. Difficulties in visualisation will also occur if the neck is flexed.
5. If possible, preoxygenate the child for a minimum of 15 seconds.
6. Hold the laryngoscope in the left hand (irrespective of handedness). While the right hand is opening the child's mouth, gently insert the laryngoscope into the right-hand corner, ensuring that the lower lip is not caught between the teeth and the blade.
7. Slide the laryngoscope blade into the mouth, sweeping the tongue to the left in the process.
8. Advance the tip of the blade. If a curved blade is used, it is usually positioned in the vallecula, the area between the back of the tongue and the base of the epiglottis. If a straight blade is used, it is usually positioned just past the epiglottis.
9. Lift the laryngoscope upwards in the line of the handle. This should lift the epiglottis out of the way and expose the glottis and vocal cords. Suction if necessary.
10. Insert the tracheal tube from the right-hand side of the mouth through the vocal cords, positioning the black marker on the tracheal tube just below the glottic opening.

11. Connect the tube to a self-inflating bag and ventilate. In older children, a catheter mount is sometimes also attached to allow greater movement of the bag. However, it should be used with caution because it increases the dead space.
12. Confirm correct tube placement (see below).
13. Secure the tube, continue ventilation and continually reassess tube position. Excessive head movement can displace the tube: the tube can be displaced further into and out of the airway by head flexion and head extension, respectively (Hartrey & Kestin, 1995).
14. Adopt a comfortable position and avoid prolonged static postures (Resuscitation Council (UK), 2011a).

Confirming correct tube placement

Misplaced, displaced or obstructed tracheal tube, which is not an uncommon complication of tracheal intubation in children, is associated with an increased risk of mortality (Gausche *et al.*, 2000; Katz & Falk, 2001). Unfortunately, no single method can be totally relied upon to detect oesophageal intubation (Andersen & Hald, 1989; Andersen & Schultz-Lebahn, 1994; Kelly *et al.*, 1998).

It is important to confirm correct tube placement as follows:

- Observe the tracheal tube passing through the vocal cords.
- Observe for mist in the tube during the expiratory phase of ventilation.
- Look for bilateral and symmetrical chest movement.
- Auscultate the chest over the axillae for breath sounds, and listen over the stomach – breath sounds should be absent over the upper abdomen (Andersen & Schultz-Lebahn, 1994).
- Auscultate over the stomach – there should be an absence of sounds of air entry during ventilation.
- Check the end-tidal carbon dioxide level – after six ventilations, a positive colour change or the presence of an exhaled carbon dioxide waveform confirms the position of the tube (Bhende *et al.*, 1992). However, this method may not be helpful during a cardiac arrest because the absence of a positive colour change or an exhaled carbon dioxide waveform does not necessarily equate with oesophageal intubation – limited pulmonary blood flow can result in undetectable exhaled carbon

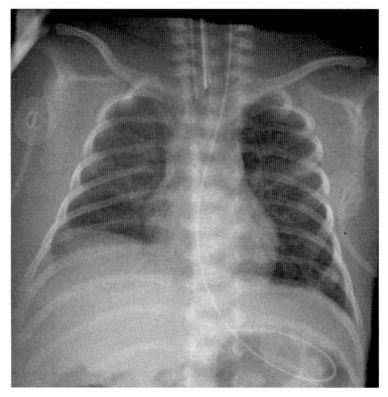

Fig. 5.14 Chest X-ray of a 1-month-old child showing a satisfactory position of the endotracheal and nasogastric tubes. ECG monitoring electrodes are also present. (The author is grateful to Dr G Pearson for his assistance.)

dioxide despite correct tracheal tube placement (Bhende & Thompson, 1995).

- Request a check chest X-ray – the tracheal tube should be in the mid-trachea, with the tip at the level of the second or third thoracic vertebra (Biarent *et al.*, 2010) (Fig. 5.14).

If in doubt, take it out.

Ineffective ventilation following tracheal intubation

Ventilation may not be established effectively after intubation, or if it is, it may become ineffective after a variable period. The main causes of this can be described by the acronym DOPES (Biarent *et al.*, 2010):

- **D**isplaced tube – either into pharynx or oesophagus, or right or left main bronchus
- **O**bstructed tube – vomit, blood, secretions or a kinked tube
- **P**neumothorax
- **E**quipment failure
- **S**tomach

These problems should be recognised and diagnosed by the checks that routinely follow intubation.

> The most common cause of failure to ventilate is improper positioning of the head and chin.

Principles of oxygen delivery and ventilation

Mouth-to-mouth ventilation has been discussed in Chapter 4. Mouth-to-mask ventilation and ventilation with a bag-valve-mask device will now be described.

Mouth-to-mask ventilation (pocket mask)

A well-fitting pocket mask used by trained rescuers is an effective method of ventilation. The standard adult pocket mask can be used in older children; in infants, it can be used upside down (Advanced Life Support Group, 2011). A paediatric pocket mask is also available.

Pocket masks are transparent, thus enabling the prompt detection of any vomit or blood in the airway. Some have a nipple for the attachment of supplementary oxygen. A one-way valve directs the child's expired air away from the rescuer.

Method

1. Move the bed away from the wall and remove the backrest if applicable. (If the child is in a cot or resuscitaire, ensure easy access.) Ensure the brakes are on.
2. Position yourself at the top of the bed facing the child, with your feet in a walk/stand position.

3. If it is available, attach oxygen to the nipple at a flow rate of 10 L per minute. This will allow the delivery of up to 50% oxygen (Lawrence & Sivaneswaran, 1985).
4. Ensure the child is supine and tilt the head back. A pillow under the head and shoulders can help to maintain this position.
5. Apply the mask to the face, pressing down with the thumbs.
6. Lift the chin into the mask by applying pressure behind the angles of the jaw.
7. Ventilate the patient with sufficient air to cause a visible chest rise. Observe for rise and fall of the chest.
8. Adopt a comfortable position for ventilation and avoid static postures.

Principles of bag-valve-mask ventilation

The face mask
Face masks come in a variety of different shapes, sizes and materials. For infants, the popular circular masks (Fig. 5.15) are generally preferred, the advantages of which include:

- A soft-cushioned rim that will conform to the contour of the baby's face, making it easier to form the seal that is essential for effective lung inflation
- Being made of transparent silicone so that secretions, etc. can be easily seen
- Minimal dead space

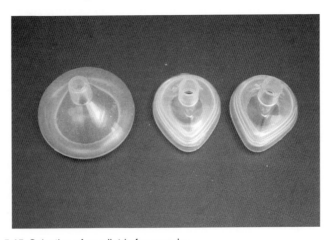

Fig. 5.15 Selection of paediatric face masks.

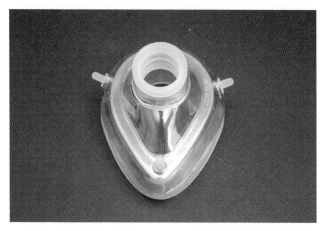

Fig. 5.16 The triangularly shaped mask recommended for older children.

Rigid triangular masks are not recommended as they are more prone to air leakage. In older children, the traditional triangularly shaped mask (Fig. 5.16) is recommended. It is important to ensure that the soft-cushioned rim is adequately inflated.

When choosing a mask, ensure that it is of an appropriate size, will fit snugly over both the mouth and the nose, but will neither cause pressure on the eyes nor create an air leak by over-riding the chin.

The self-inflating bag

There are a number of different makes of self-inflating bag available, but they all work on the same principle. Personnel using this device ought to be familiar with its structure and function. The self-inflating bag (Fig. 5.17) consists of the following components:

- *The bag* – different bag sizes are available. The 500 mL bag (Fig. 5.17) should be used for the resuscitation of infants and small children. It will reinflate by recoil after being squeezed even if no gas is entering. The 1500 mL (adult) bag (Fig. 5.18) is generally only used in older children. However, it could be used (with extreme care) in infants (Terndrup *et al.*, 1989). The 250 mL (neonatal) bag is considered too small for infant resuscitation (Field *et al.*, 1986).

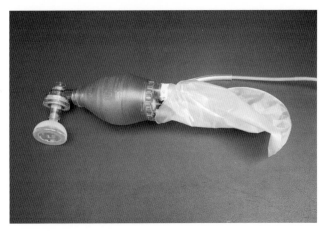

Fig. 5.17 Paediatric self-inflating bag.

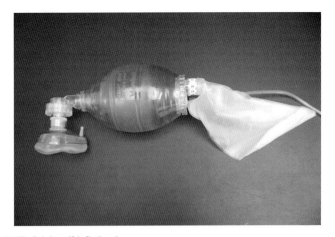

Fig. 5.18 Adult self-inflating bag.

- *The air inlet* – oxygen is sucked through the air inlet if the oxygen reservoir bag is full and attached. If it is not attached, air will be sucked through.
- *The oxygen inlet* – oxygen is delivered to the bag here at a recommended rate of 15 L per minute (as long as the oxygen tubing is connected and the flowmeter is turned on!).
- *The reservoir bag* – with an oxygen flow rate of 15 L per minute, this will increase the oxygen concentration delivered to the

baby to almost 100%. Oxygen is allowed to fill the reservoir during expiration, enabling rapid refilling of the bag.

- *The patient outlet* – this connects directly to the face mask or the tracheal tube adapter.
- *The outlet valve* – this is situated between the bag and the patient outlet. It opens when the bag is squeezed, allowing gas through to the child.
- *The pressure relief valve* – this is situated between the bag and outlet valve. It opens at about 30–40 cmH$_2$O, preventing very high pressures being generated that could cause a pneumothorax. However, there must be an override feature so that high pressures can be generated if required in order to achieve chest rise (Hirschman & Kravath, 1982). Higher pressures may be required if there is upper or lower airway obstruction or if there is poor lung compliance – in these situations, a pressure relief valve may prevent the delivery of a sufficient tidal volume (Finer *et al.*, 1986).
- *The inlet valve* – this is situated between the bag and the air inlet. It allows air to enter the bag during refilling but prevents its exit during squeezing.
- *The oxygen reservoir valve* – this allows excess oxygen to escape, so there is no problem with an oxygen flow rate of 15 L per minute

Although the bag-valve-mask device allows the delivery of higher concentrations of oxygen, its use by one person requires considerable skill, and the technique may in fact be ineffective when undertaken by one person. A two-person technique is thus recommended (Resuscitation Council (UK), 2011a), with one person to open the airway and ensure a good seal with the mask, while the other squeezes the bag (Fig. 5.19). An oxygen reservoir bag should ideally be used as this will enable the delivery of high concentrations of oxygen.

Method

1. Move the bed away from the wall and remove the backrest if applicable. Ensure the bed's brakes are on.
2. Position yourself at the top of the bed facing the child, with your feet in a walk/stand position.
3. Select an appropriately sized mask. This should comfortably cover the mouth and nose; it should *not* cover the eyes or

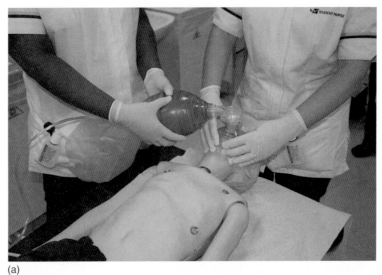

(a)

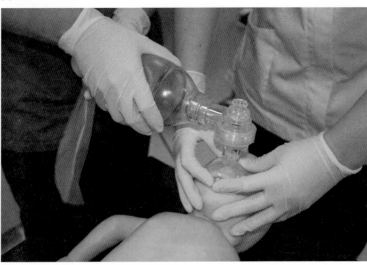

(b)

Fig. 5.19 The two-person technique for using a self-inflating bag.

override the chin. It should be transparent, thus enabling a prompt detection of any vomit or blood in the airway. It should also have a soft pliable edge to facilitate achieving a good seal with the face.

4. Select an appropriately sized bag.
5. Ensure that the oxygen reservoir bag is attached, and connect the oxygen at a flow rate of 10–15 L per minute (Finer *et al.*, 1986). This will usually achieve an inspired oxygen concentration of approximately 85% (Resuscitation Council (UK), 2011a).
6. Ensure the child is supine. The first rescuer should tilt the head back and apply the mask to the face, pressing down on it with the thumbs. The chin should then be lifted into the mask by applying pressure behind the angles of the jaw. An open airway and an adequate seal between the face and the mask should now be achieved. For a child, a pillow under the head and shoulders can help to maintain this position. In an infant and smaller child, a rolled-up blanket under the shoulders may help.
7. Ask your colleague, who should be positioned to the side of the bed, to slowly squeeze the bag-valve device (not the oxygen reservoir bag) with sufficient air to cause a visible rise of the chest (Fig. 5.19).
8. Observe for rise and fall of the chest. If the chest does not rise, recheck the patency of the airway. Slight readjustment may be all that is required.
9. Adopt a comfortable position for ventilation and avoid static postures. Supporting your weight by resting your elbows on the bed may help.

If ventilation is judged to be ineffective, recheck airway patency and the seal between the face and the mask, and consider equipment failure. In each case, take the appropriate action. If the lungs are known to be stiff, a higher inflation pressure can be tried by disabling the pressure relief valve.

Gastric inflation

Unless the child's airway is secured with a tracheal tube, ventilation carries a high risk of gastric inflation, regurgitation of gastric contents and pulmonary aspiration. Gastric inflation can also limit effective ventilation. There is an increased risk of gastric inflation when:

- Inflation pressures and volumes are high
- The head and neck are not aligned
- The airway is not patent
- The oesophageal sphincter is incompetent

To minimise the risk of gastric inflation, the following are recommended:

- Gently squeeze the bag.
- Deliver a tidal volume to achieve chest rise.
- Ensure a patent airway.

If gastric distension develops, the stomach should be decompressed with a nasogastric tube (American Academy of Pediatrics, 2000)

Importance of avoiding hyperventilation

Healthcare practitioners often hyperventilate during resuscitation, but hyperventilation can be harmful because it increases intrathoracic pressure, decreases cerebral and coronary perfusion, and leads to poorer survival rates in animals and adults (Aufderheide & Lurie, 2004; Aufderheide *et al.*, 2004; O'Neill & Deakin, 2007).

To help achieve normoventilation during resuscitation (Biarent *et al.*, 2010):

- Press the bag just sufficiently to achieve a rise of the chest.
- Follow a ratio of 15 chest compressions to 2 ventilations.
- Once the child is intubated, continue positive-pressure ventilation at a rate of 12–20 ventilations per minute (higher rates in infants) without interrupting chest compressions.

Principles of oxygenation administration

During initial resuscitation, oxygen should be administered at the highest concentration (i.e. 100%; Biarent *et al.*, 2010). However, following the return of spontaneous circulation, supplementary oxygen should be guided by pulse oximetry, with the aim

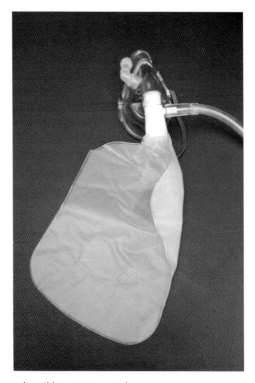

Fig. 5.20 Non-rebreathing oxygen mask.

of achieving an arterial oxygen saturation (Sao_2) of 94–98% (Seguin *et al.*, 2000; Van de Louw *et al.*, 2001; Resuscitation Council (UK), 2011a).

Using a non-rebreathing oxygen mask

The non-rebreathing oxygen mask (Fig. 5.20) enables the delivery of high concentrations of oxygen and is recommended for use in critically ill children (Resuscitation Council (UK), 2011a).

Description
The non-rebreathing mask (sometimes called a Hudson mask) with an oxygen reservoir bag has a one-way valve that diverts the oxygen flow into the reservoir bag during expiration. The contents of the reservoir bag, together with the high-flow oxygen, results in minimal entrainment of air and an inspired oxygen concentration of approximately 85% (Gwinnutt, 2006). The valve

also prevents the patient's exhaled gases from entering the reservoir bag. Use of the oxygen reservoir bag helps to increase the inspired oxygen concentration by preventing oxygen loss during inspiration (Leach, 2009).

Some non-rebreather masks have elasticated earloop bands. As these eliminate the need to move the child's head, they are frequently used in accident and emergency departments for trauma patients.

Prior to use

It is important to ensure that a sufficient oxygen flow rate is used so that the oxygen reservoir bag does not collapse during inspiration (Resuscitation Council (UK), 2011a). An oxygen flow rate of 12–15 L per minute is recommended (Gwinnutt, 2006).

To ensure that the mask is functioning correctly and is effectively used, it is important to follow the manufacturer's recommendations for simple basic checks prior to use (Intersurgical, 2003; Fig. 5.21).

Procedure

- Encourage the child to adopt an upright position to maximise breathing.
- Request that pulse oximetry is commenced.
- Explain the procedure to the child and the parents.
- Attach the oxygen tubing to the oxygen source.
- Set the oxygen flow rate to 12–15 L per minute (Gwinnutt, 2006).
- Occlude the valve between the mask and the oxygen reservoir bag (Fig. 5.21) and check that the reservoir bag is filling up. Remove the finger.
- Squeeze the oxygen reservoir bag (Fig. 5.21) to check the patency of the valve between the mask and the reservoir bag. If the valve is working correctly, it will be possible to empty the reservoir bag; if the reservoir bag does not empty, discard it and select another mask (Smith, 2003).
- Again occlude the valve between the mask and the oxygen reservoir bag (Fig. 5.21), allowing the reservoir bag to fill up.
- Place the mask with a filled oxygen reservoir bag on the child's face, ensuring a secure fit.

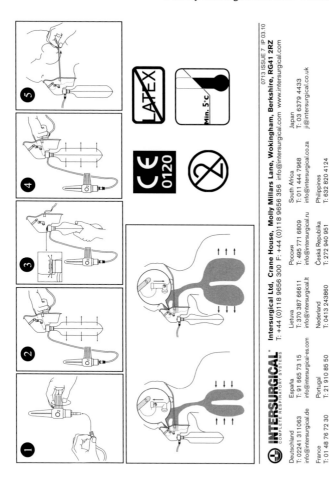

0713 ISSUE 7 IP 03.10

INTERSURGICAL ®
COMPLETE RESPIRATORY SYSTEMS

Intersurgical Ltd, Crane House, Molly Millars Lane, Wokingham, Berkshire, RG41 2RZ
T: +44 (0)118 9656 300 F: +44 (0)118 9656 356 info@intersurgical.com www.intersurgical.com

Deutschland
T: 02241 311063
info@intersurgical.de

France
T: 01 48 76 72 30
info@intersurgical.fr

España
T: 91 665 73 15
info@intersurgical-es.com

Portugal
T: 21 910 85 50
info@intersurgical.pt

Lietuva
T: 370 387 66611
info@intersurgical.lt

Nederland
T: 0413 243860
info@intersurgical.nl

Россия
T: 495 771 6809
info@intersurgical.ru

Česká Republika
T: 272 940 951
info@intersurgical.cz

South Africa
T: 011 444 7968
info@intersurgical.co.za

Philippines
T: 632 820 4124
info@intersurgical.ph

Japan
T: 03 6379 4433
ji@intersurgical.co.uk

(a)

Fig. 5.21 Preparing to use a non-rebreathing oxygen mask. Reproduced with kind permission of Intersurgical.

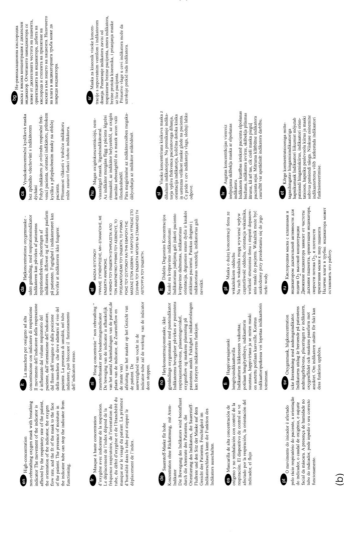

en High-concentration
non-rebreathing oxygen mask with breathing indicator The movement of the indicator is affected by the respiratory rate of the patient, the orientation of the indicator, the oxygen flow rate, and the fit of the mask to the face of the patient. The presence of moisture in the indicator tube can stop the indicator from functioning.

es Mascarilla de alta concentración de oxígeno y no reinhalación con control de la respiración. El dispositivo de control se ve afectado por la respiración, la orientación del indicador, el flujo

pt O movimento do inalador é afectado pelo ritmo respiratório do paciente, a orientação do indicador, o caudal de oxigénio, e ajuste facial da máscara. A presença de humidade no tubo do indicador, pode impedir o seu correcto funcionamento.

de Sauerstoff-Maske für hohe Konzentration ohne Rückatmung, mit Atemhilfe. Die Bewegung des Indikators wird beeinflusst durch die Atemfrequenz des Patienten, die Orientierung des Indikators, die Sauerstoff-Flußrate und den Sitz der Maske auf dem Gesicht des Patienten. Feuchtigkeit im Indikatorschlauch kann die Funktion des Indikators ausschalten.

it La maschera per ossigeno ad alta concentrazione senza respirazione. Il movimento dell'indicatore della respirazione è influenzato dal volume respiratorio del paziente, dall'orientazione dell'indicatore, dal flusso dell'ossigeno e dalla posizione della maschera che deve adattarsi al viso del paziente. La presenza di umidità, nel tubo dell'indicatore, può bloccare il funzionamento dell'indicatore stesso.

nl Hoog concentratie "non rebreathing" zuurstofmasker met beademingsindicator. De beweging van de indicator is afhankelijk van het aantal Ademhalingen van de patient,de plaats van de indicator, de Zuurstofflow en de mate van afsluiting van het masker op het Gezicht van de patient. De aanwezigheid van vocht in de indicator-tube zal de werking van de indicator doen stoppen.

el ΜΑΣΚΑ ΘΕΥΓΟΝΟΥ ΥΨΗΛΗΣ ΣΥΓΚΕΝΤΡΩΣΗΣ ΜΗ-ΕΠΑΝΑΠΝΟΗΣ, ΜΕ ΕΝΔΕΙΚΤΗ ΑΝΑΠΝΟΗΣ. Η ΚΙΝΗΣΗ ΤΟΥ ΕΝΔΕΙΚΤΗ ΕΠΗΡΕΑΖΕΤΑΙ ΑΠΟ ΤΟΝ ΑΝΑΠΝΕΥΣΤΙΚΟ ΡΥΘΜΟ ΤΟΥ ΑΣΘΕΝΟΥΣ, ΤΟ ΠΡΟΣΑΝΑΤΟΛΙΣΜΟ ΤΟΥ ΕΝΔΕΙΚΤΗ, ΤΟ ΡΥΘΜΟ ΡΟΗΣ ΤΟΥ ΟΞΥΓΟΝΟΥ ΚΑΙ ΤΗΝ ΕΦΑΡΜΟΓΗ ΤΗΣ ΜΑΣΚΑΣ ΣΤΟΝ ΑΣΘΕΝΗ. Η ΠΑΡΟΥΣΙΑ ΥΓΡΑΣΙΑΣ ΣΤΟ ΣΩΛΗΝΑ ΤΟΥ ΕΝΔΕΙΚΤΗ ΜΠΟΡΕΙ ΝΑ ΣΤΑΜΑΤΗΣΕΙ ΤΗ ΛΕΙΤΟΥΡΓΙΑ ΤΟΥ ΕΝΔΕΙΚΤΗ.

fi Happivaraajamaski hengitysindikaattorilla Indikaattorin liikkeeseen vaikuttaa potilaan hengitystiheys, indikaattorin suuntaus, happivirtaus ja se miten maski on asetettu potilaan kasvoille. Kosteus indikaattoriputkessa voi lopettaa indikaattorin toiminnan.

sv Oxygenmask, högkoncentration icke återandnings med andningsindikator. Indikatorns utslag är beroende på patientens andningsfrekvens, placeringen av indikatorn, oxygenflödet och maskens passform mot dess funktion uppföras.

ru Кислородная маска с вдыханием и индикатором дыхательной активности для подачи О₂ высокой концентрации. Движение индикатора зависит от частоты дыхания пациента, ориентации индикатора, скорости потока О₂, и плотности прилегания маски к лицу пациента. Наличие влаги в трубке индикатора может остановить его работу.

da Højkoncentrations oxygenmaske - uden genånding, med respirationsindikator Indikatorens kan påvirkes af patientens respirationstilstand, placeringen af indikatoren, ilttilførsel og af maskens passform på patientens. Fugtighed i indikatorrøret kan bevirke at indikatorens ikke fungerer.

cs Vysokokoncentrační kyslíková maska bez zpětného vdechování s indikátorem dýchání Pohyb indikátoru je ovlivněn respirační frekvencí pacienta, orientací indikátoru, průtokem kyslíku a přizpůsobením masky na obličej pacienta. Přítomnost vlhkosti v trubičce indikátoru může zastavit funkci tohoto indikátoru.

hu Magas oxigénkoncentrációjú, nem-visszalégző maszk, légzésindikátorral. Az indikátor mozgását függ a páciens légzési ritmusától, az indikátor helyzetétől, az oxigén áramlási sebességétől és a maszk arcon való illeszkedésétől. Pára megjelenése az indikátorcsőben megakadályozhatja az indikátor működését.

sl Visoko koncentrirana kisikova maska z dihalnim indikatorjem. Na premikanje indikatorja vpliva frekvenca pacientovega dihanja, orientacija indikatorja, količina dotoka kisika ter ustreznega tesnitve maske glede na pacienta. Če pride v cev indikatorja vlaga, slednji lahko odpove.

lt Didelės Deguonies Koncentracijos Kaukė su kvėpavimo indikatoriumi Indikatoriaus judėjimą gali įtakoti paciento kvėpavimo dažnumas, indikatoriaus orientacija, deguonies srauto dydis ir kaukės atitikimas pacientui. Patekus drėgmei į indikatoriaus vamzdelį, indikatorius gali neveikti.

lv Augstas koncentrācijas vairāki neelpojama skābekļa maska ar elpošanas indikatoru. Indikatora kustība ietekmē pacienta elpošanas biežums, indikatora ievirze, skābekļa plūsmas ātrums, kā arī, cik cieši maska piegul pacienta sejai. Mitruma klātbūtne indikatora cauruļlītē var apstādināt indikatora darbību.

et Kõrge kontsentratsiooniga mittetagasihingatav hingamisindikaatoriga hapnikumask Indikaatori liikumist mõjutab patsiendi hingamissagedus, indikaatori orientatsioon, hapniku pealevoolu kiirus ja maski sobivus patsiendi näoga. Niiskuse esinemine indikaatoritorus võib katkestada indikaatori funktsioneerimise.

bg Не-реинхалационна кислородна маска с висока концентрация с дихателен индикатор. Отчитането на индикатора се влияе от дихателната честота на пациента, ориентацията на индикатора, дебита на кислорода и степента на прилягане на маската към лицето на пациента. Наличието на влага в индикаторната тръба може да повреди индикатора.

cf Маска за кислени, висок концентрация с непропускливост и индикатор на дишане. Помрачене индикатора зависи од респираторне брзине пацијента, смера индикатора, брзине протока кислеоника, и прианјања маске уз лице пацијента. Присуство влаге у цеви индикатора може да узрокује прекид рада индикатора.

(b)

Fig. 5.21 *continued*

- Adjust the oxygen flow rate sufficiently to ensure that the reservoir bag deflates by approximately one-third with each breath (Smith, 2003).
- Reassure the child.
- Closely monitor the child's vital signs. In particular, assess the patient's response to the oxygen therapy, e.g. respiratory rate, mechanics of breathing, colour, oxygen saturation levels and level of consciousness. Arterial blood gas analysis may need to be performed.
- Discontinue or reduce the inspired oxygen concentration as appropriate following advice from a suitably qualified practitioner

(Source: Intersurgical, 2003)

Respiratory rate indicator

Some masks have a respiratory rate indicator to help the health-care practitioner to monitor the patient's respiratory rate. This indicator can be affected by (Intersurgical, 2003):

- The patient's respiratory rate
- The orientation of the indicator
- The oxygen flow rate
- The fit of the mask to the patient's face
- The presence of moisture in the indicator tube – this can actually stop the indicator working

Note that the respiratory rate indicator should only be used as a guide and should not replace close monitoring of the patient's breathing.

Summary

Effective airway management and ventilation are essential aspects of paediatric resuscitation. Relevant anatomy and physiology, causes and recognition of airway obstruction have been discussed, as have simple techniques to open and clear the airway, together with the principles of cricoid pressure. The roles of oropharyngeal, nasopharyngeal and laryngeal mask airways have been discussed. The procedure for tracheal intubation and the principles of ventilation and oxygenation have been highlighted.

References

Abernethy, J.L., Allan, P.L. & Drummond, G.B. (1990) Ultrasound assessment of the position of the tongue during induction of anaesthesia. *British Journal of Anaesthesia*, **65**, 744–748.

Advanced Life Support Group (2011) *Advanced Paediatric Life Support*, 5th edn. Wiley Blackwell, Oxford.

American Academy of Pediatrics (1997) *Pediatric Advanced Life Support*. American Heart Association, Dallas, TX.

American Academy of Pediatrics (2000) *Pediatric Education for Prehospital Professionals*. Jones & Bartlett, Sudbury, MA.

Andersen, K. & Hald, A. (1989) Assessing the position of the tracheal tube: the reliability of different methods. *Anaesthesia*, **44**, 984–985.

Andersen, K. & Schultz-Lebahn, T. (1994) Oesophageal intubation can be undetected by auscultation of the chest. *Acta Anaesthesiologica Scandinavica*, **38**, 580–582.

Aufderheide, T. & Lurie, K. (2004) Death by hyperventilation: a common and lifethreatening problem during cardiopulmonary resuscitation. *Critical Care Medicine*, **32**, S345–S351.

Aufderheide, T., Sigurdsson, G., Pirrallo R *et al.* (2004) Hyperventilation induced hypotension during cardiopulmonary resuscitation. *Circulation*, **109**, 1960–1965.

Bhende, M. & Thompson, A. (1995) Evaluation of an end-tidal CO2 detector during pediatric cardiopulmonary resuscitation. *Pediatrics*, **95**, 395–399.

Bhende, M., Thompson, A., Cook, D. & Saville, A. (1992) Validity of a disposable end-tidal CO2 detector in verifying endotracheal tube placement in infants and children. *Annals of Emergency Medicine*, **21**, 142–145.

Biarent, D., Bingham, R., Christoph, E. *et al.* (2010) European Resuscitation Council Guidelines for Resuscitation Section 6. Paediatric life support (2010). *Resuscitation*, **81**, 1364–1388.

Blevin, A., McDouall, S., Rechner, J. *et al.* (2009) A comparison of the laryngeal mask airway with the facemask and oropharyngeal airway for manual ventilation by first responders in children. *Anaesthesia*, **64**, 1312–1316.

Cote, C. & Todres, I. (1990) The paediatric airway. In: *A Practice of Anaesthesia for Infants and Children* (eds C. Cote, J. Ryan, I. Todres & N. Groudsouzian), 2nd edn. WB Saunders, Philadelphia.

Cross, K., Tizard, J. & Trythall, D. (1957) The gaseous metabolism of the newborn infant. *Acta Paediatrica*, **46**, 265–285.

Deakers, T., Reynolds, G., Stretton, M. & Newth, C. (1994) Cuffed endotracheal tubes in pediatric intensive care. *Journal of Pediatrics*, **125**, 57–62.

Field, D., Milner, A. & Hipkin, I. (1986) Efficiency of manual resuscitators at birth. *Archives of Disease in Childhood*, **61**, 300–302.

Finer, N., Barrington, K., Al-Fadley, F. & Peters, K. (1986) Limitations of self-inflating resuscitators. *Pediatrics*, **77**, 417–420.

Friesen, R.M., Duncan, P. & Tweed, W. (1982) Appraisal of pediatric cardiopulmonary resuscitation. *Canadian Medical Association Journal*, **126**, 1055–1058.

Gausche, M., Lewis, R., Stratton, S. *et al.* (2000) Effect of out-of-hospital pediatric endotracheal intubation on survival and neurological outcome: a controlled clinical trial. *JAMA*, **283**, 783–790.

Gwinnutt, C. (2006) *Clinical Anaesthesia*, 2nd edn. Blackwell Publishing, Oxford.

Harnett, M., Kinirons, B., Heffernan, A. *et al.* (2000) Airway complications in infants: comparison of laryngeal mask airway and the facemask-oral airway. *Canadian Journal of Anaesthesia*, **47**, 315–318.

Hartrey, R. & Kestin, I. (1995) Movement of oral and nasal tracheal tubes as a result of changes in head and neck position. *Anaesthesia*, **50**, 682–687.

Hartsilver, E. & Vanner, R. (2000) Airway obstruction with cricoid pressure. *Anaesthesia*, **55**, 208–211.

Hirschman, A. & Kravath, R. (1982) Venting vs. ventilating: a danger of manual resuscitation bags. *Chest*, **82**, 369–370.

Hugdel, D.W. & Hendricks, C. (1988) Palate and hypopharynx: sites of inspiratory narrowing of the upper airway during sleep. *American Review of Respiratory Diseases*, **138**, 1542–1547.

Intersurgical (2003) *Non-rebreathing Mask Product Literature*. Intersurgical, Wokingham.

Jevon P (2009) *Advanced Cardiac Life Support*, 2nd edn. Wiley Blackwell, Oxford.

Katz, S. & Falk, J. (2001) Misplaced endotracheal tubes by paramedics in an urban emergency medical services system. *Annals of Emergency Medicine*, **37**, 32–37.

Kaye, K., Frascone, R. & Held, T. (2003) Prehospital rapid-sequence intubation: a pilot training program. *Prehospital Emergency Care*, **7**, 235–240.

Kelly, J., Eynon, C., Kaplan, J. *et al.* (1998) Use of tube condensation as an indicator of endotracheal tube placement. *Annals of Emergency Medicine*, **31**, 575–578.

Khine, H., Cordrry, D., Kettrick, R. *et al.* (1997) Comparison of cuffed and uncuffed endotracheal tubes in young children in general anaesthesia. *Anesthesiology*, **86**, 627–631.

Lawrence, P. & Sivaneswaran, N. (1985) Ventilation during cardiopulmonary resuscitation: which method? *Medical Journal of Australia*, **143**, 443–446.

Leach R (2009) *Acute and Critical Care Medicine at a Glance*, 2nd edn. Blackwell Wiley, Oxford.

Luten, R., Wears, R., Broselow, J. *et al.* (1992) Length-based endotracheal tube and emergency equipment in pediatrics. *Annals of Emergency Medicine*, **21**, 900–904.

Mansell, A., Bryan, C. & Levison, H. (1972) Airway closure in children. *Journal of Applied Physiology*, **33**, 711–714.

Mhanna, M., Zamel, Y., Tichy, C. & Super, D. (2002) The "air leak" test around the endotracheal tube, as a predictor of postextubation stridor, is age dependent in children. *Critical Care Medicine*, **30**, 2639–2643.

Moynihan, R., Brock-Utne, J., Archer, J. *et al.* (1993) The effect of cricoid pressure on preventing gastric inflation in infants and children. *Anesthesiology*, **78**, 652–656.

Newth, C., Rachman, B., Patel, N. & Hammer, J. (2004) The use of cuffed versus uncuffed endotracheal tubes in pediatric intensive care. *Journal of Pediatrics*, **144**, 333–337.

O'Neill, J. & Deakin, C. (2007) Do we hyperventilate cardiac arrest patients? *Resuscitation*, **73**, 82–85.

Park, C., Bahk, J., Ahn, W. *et al.* (2001) The laryngeal mask airway in infants and children. *Canadian Journal of Anaesthesia*, **48**, 413–417.

Rechner, J., Loach, V., Ali, M. *et al.* (2007) A comparison of the laryngeal mask airway with facemask and oropharyngeal airway for manual ventilation by critical care nurses in children. *Anaesthesia*, **62**, 790–795.

Resuscitation Council (UK) (2011a) *Paediatric Immediate Life Support*, 2nd edn. Resuscitation Council (UK), London.

Resuscitation Council (UK) (2011b) *European Paediatric Life Support*, 3rd edn. Resuscitation Council (UK), London.

Ruben, H.M., Elam, J.O., & Ruben, A.M. (1961) Investigation of upper airway problems in resuscitation. Studies of pharyngeal X-rays and performance by lay men. *Anesthesiology*, **22**, 271–279.

Salem, M., Joseph, N., Heyman, H. *et al.* (1985) Cricoid compression is effective in obliterating the esophageal lumen in the presence of a nasogastric tube. *Anesthesiology*, **63**, 443–446.

Seguin, P., Le Rouzo, A., Tanguy, M. *et al.* (2000) Evidence for the need of bedside accuracy of pulse oximetry in an intensive care unit. *Critical Care Medicine*, **28**, 703–706.

Smith, G. (2003) *ALERT*, 2nd edn. University of Portsmouth, Portsmouth.

Tendrup, T., Kanter, R. & Cherry, R. (1989) A comparison of infant ventilation methods performed by pre-hospital personnel. *Annals of Emergency Medicine*, **18**, 607–611.

Van de Louw, A., Cracco, C., Cerf, C. *et al.* (2001) Accuracy of pulse oximetry in the intensive care unit. *Intensive Care Medicine*, **27**, 1606–1613.

Walker, R., Ravi, R. & Haylett, K. (2010) Effect of cricoid force on airway calibre in children: a bronchoscopic assessment. *British Journal of Anaesthesia*, **104**, 71–74.

Wang, H., Sweeney, T., O'Connor, R. & Rubinstein, H. (2001) Failed prehospital intubations: an analysis of emergency department courses and outcomes. *Prehospital Emergency Care*, **5**, 134–141.

Wang, H., Kupas, D., Paris, P. *et al.* (2003) Multivariate predictors of failed prehospital endotracheal intubation. *Academic Emergency Medicine*, **10**, 717–724.

Weiss, M., Dullenkopf, A., Fischer, J. *et al.* (2009) Prospective randomized controlled multi-centre trial of cuffed or uncuffed endotracheal tubes in small children. *British Journal of Anaesthesia*, **103**, 867–873.

Wittenborg, M., Gyepes, M. & Crocker, D. (1967) Tracheal dynamics in infants with respiratory distress, stridor, and collapsing trachea. *Radiology*, **88**, 653–662.

Chapter 6

ECG Recognition and Management of Cardiac Arrhythmias

Introduction

Life-threatening cardiac arrhythmias in children usually result from rather than cause acute illness (Resuscitation Council (UK), 2011). ECG monitoring is nevertheless still an important aspect of paediatric advanced life support. Once the presenting ECG rhythm has been identified, the appropriate treatment can then be administered. Poor technique can, however, lead to an inaccurate ECG trace and mistaken diagnosis. A sound knowledge of the principles of ECG monitoring is therefore paramount.

An understanding of the principles of ECG recognition is also important. It will enable the identification of abnormal ECG rhythms that may compromise cardiac output, precede or be associated with cardiac arrest, or complicate recovery after successful cardiopulmonary resuscitation (CPR). An understanding of the basic principles of ECG recognition is therefore essential. It is also important to understand the management of cardiac arrhythmias.

The aim of this chapter is for readers to understand the principles of ECG monitoring and the management of cardiac arrhythmias.

Paediatric Advanced Life Support: A Practical Guide for Nurses, Second Edition. Phil Jevon.
© 2012 Phil Jevon. Published 2012 by Blackwell Publishing Ltd.

Learning objectives

At the end of this chapter, the reader will be able to:

- Describe the conduction system of the heart
- Describe the ECG and its relation to cardiac contraction
- Describe a suggested ECG electrode placement for ECG monitoring
- State the problems that can be encountered with ECG monitoring
- Discuss the management of cardiac arrhythmias
- Outline the treatment of bradycardia and sinus tachycardia
- Outline the recognition and treatment of supraventricular tachycardia (SVT) and ventricular tachycardia (VT)

The conduction system of the heart

The heart possesses specialised muscle cells that initiate and conduct electrical impulses resulting in myocardial contraction. This conduction system (Fig. 6.1) comprises the following:

- Sinus node (also known as the sinoatrial node)
- Atrioventricular node or junction
- Bundle of His
- Bundle branches (right and left)
- Purkinje fibres

Nervous control of the heart rate

The sinus node normally acts as the pacemaker for myocardial contraction, the rate at which it fires being dependent upon the autonomic nervous system:

- *Parasympathetic or vagus nerve* – an increase in activity slows the heart rate, while a decrease in activity speeds the heart rate up. Atropine blocks the vagus nerve, causing an increase in heart rate.
- *Sympathetic nerve* – this prepares the body for 'fight or flight' and will result in an increase in heart rate and an increase in the force of myocardial contraction.

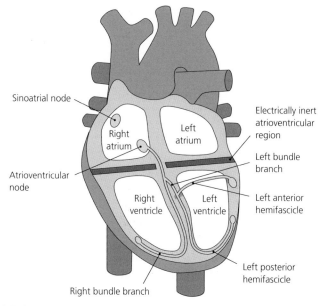

Fig. 6.1 Conduction system of the heart. Reproduced from Morris, F. *et al.*, *ABC of Clinical Electrocardiography*, 2nd edn, copyright 2008, with permission of Blackwell Publishing.

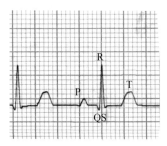

Fig. 6.2 The ECG and cardiac contraction.

The ECG and its relation to cardiac contraction

Figure 6.2 depicts the ECG and how it relates to cardiac contraction. The explanation of the PQRST complex and how it is associated with cardiac activity is as follows (Jevon, 2009):

1. The sinus node fires, and the electrical impulse spreads across the atria causing atrial contraction (the P wave).

2. On arriving at the atrioventricular node, the impulse is delayed to allow the atria time to fully contract and eject blood into the ventricles. This brief period of absent electrical activity is represented on the ECG by a straight (isoelectric) line between the end of the P wave and the beginning of the QRS complex.
3. The impulse is then conducted to the ventricles through the bundle of His, right and left bundle branches and Purkinje fibres, causing ventricular depolarisation and contraction (the QRS complex).
4. The ventricles then repolarise (the T wave).

Sinus rhythm is the normal rhythm (Fig. 6.3), indicating that the impulse is initiated by the sinoatrial node at a normal rate for the child's age and is conducted down the normal conduction pathways without being delayed.

Suggested ECG electrode placement for cardiac monitoring

During paediatric resuscitation, lead II is the best lead for cardiac monitoring. The monitor/defibrillator should be switched on,

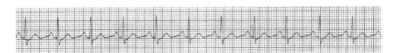

Fig. 6.3 Sinus rhythm.

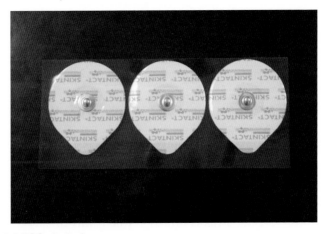

Fig. 6.4 ECG electrodes.

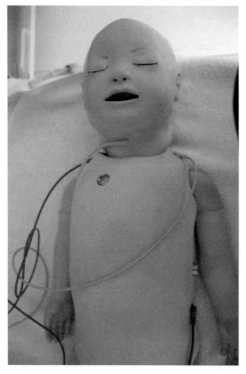

Fig. 6.5 Standard ECG electrode placement for cardiac monitoring.

lead II should be selected, and the ECG electrodes (Fig. 6.4) should be positioned as follows:

- *Red* on the right shoulder
- *Yellow* on the left shoulder
- *Green* on the left upper abdominal wall

This standard ECG electrode placement (Fig. 6.5) benefits from reduced muscle interference and will not hinder paddle placement if defibrillation is required.

In the resuscitation situation, initial ECG monitoring is sometimes established using the large adhesive defibrillation pads (see Chapter 8).

Problems encountered with ECG monitoring

Problems encountered with cardiac monitoring include the following:

- *A 'straight line' ECG trace* – check the child, monitoring the lead selected (normally lead II), ECG gain, ECG leads and electrodes. Note that asystole is rarely a straight line.
- *A poor quality ECG trace* – check all the connections and the brightness display. Ensure that the electrodes are correctly attached and are 'in date', and that the gel sponge is moist, not dry (Jevon, 2009). Ensure the skin where the electrodes are attached is dry.
- *Interference and artefacts* – poor electrode contact, child movement, CPR and electrical interference, e.g. from bedside infusion pumps, can cause the ECG trace to be 'fuzzy'. Apply the electrodes over bone rather than muscle to minimise interference (Jevon, 2009).
- *A wandering baseline* – an ECG trace that goes up and down is usually caused by movement of the child or simply by ventilation. Reposition the electrodes away from the lower ribs.
- *Small ECG complexes* – the most likely cause of small and unrecognisable ECG complexes is a technical problem. Check that the ECG gain is adequate and that appropriate ECG monitoring lead (lead II) has been selected on the monitor.
- *Incorrect heart rate display* – causes include small QRS complexes, large T waves, muscle movement and interference. Ensure that the ECG trace is reliable. It is also important to measure the heart rate manually (Resuscitation Council (UK), 2011)

Management of cardiac arrhythmias

The Resuscitation Council (UK) (2011) recommends a systematic approach to the management of cardiac arrhythmias in children (Fig. 6.6). This approach encompasses four key factors (Resuscitation Council (UK), 2011):

- *Circulation status* – present or absent
- *Clinical status* – compensated or decompensated
- *Heart rate* – bradycardia or tachycardia
- *Width of QRS complex* – narrow or broad

Circulation status

Following the ABCDE approach, quickly determine whether circulation is present (a central pulse and signs of life) or absent:

Managing the child with a cardiac arrhythmia

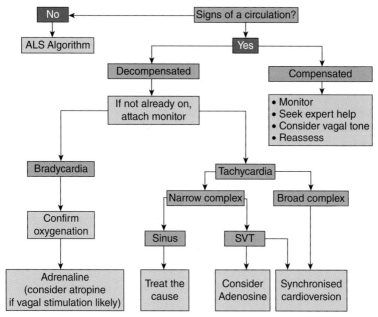

Fig. 6.6 Resuscitation Council (UK) (2011) algorithm for managing a child with a cardiac arrhythmia. ALS, advanced life support; SVT, supraventricular tachycardia. Reproduced with kind permission of the Resuscitation Council (UK).

- *Circulation present* – determine whether the child is compensated (haemodynamically stable) or decompensated (haemodynamically unstable) (Advanced Life Support Group, 2011).
- *Circulation absent* – begin CPR immediately following the Resuscitation Council (UK) guidelines for basic life support (see Chapter 4) and where appropriate advanced life support (see Chapter 8).

Clinical status

Following the ABCDE approach, determine whether the child is compensated (haemodynamically stable) or decompensated (haemodynamically unstable) (see Chapter 3) (Resuscitation Council (UK), 2011):

- *Compensated* – monitor the child and await expert help.
- *Decompensated* – monitor the child, call for expert help and if necessary start emergency treatment as described in Fig. 6.6.

Heart rate

Determine the child's heart rate by checking a central pulse. If an ECG rhythm strip is available, estimate the QRS rate by counting the number of large squares between adjacent QRS complexes and dividing it into 300; for example, the QRS rate in Fig. 6.3 is about 150 (300/2). Care should be taken if the QRS rate is irregular. Establish whether the QRS rate is normal, abnormally slow (bradycardia) or abnormally fast (tachycardia).

Bradycardia (<80 beats per minute in infants and <60 beats per minute in children)

- Causes of bradycardia (Fig. 6.7) include hypoxia, acidosis, respiratory or circulatory failure, poisoning and increased vagal tone (e.g. induced by tracheal intubation or suctioning) (Advanced Life Support Group, 2011).

Tachycardia (>180 in infants beats per minute and >160 beats per minute in children)

- Causes of sinus tachycardia (Fig. 6.8) include shock, e.g. fluid loss, haemorrhage or anaphylaxis, pain, pyrexia and anxiety (a normal physiological response).

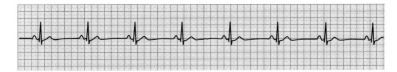

Fig. 6.7 Sinus bradycardia.

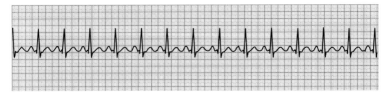

Fig. 6.8 Sinus tachycardia.

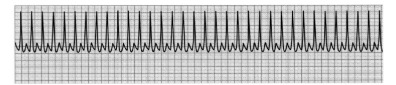

Fig. 6.9 Supraventricular tachycardia.

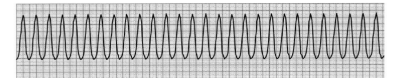

Fig. 6.10 Ventricular tachycardia.

- Tachycardia can also be due to a tachyarrhythmia: SVT (Fig. 6.9) or less commonly VT (Fig. 6.10). Treatment includes following the ABCDE approach and establishing whether child is compensated or decompensated; for the latter, chemical or electrical cardioversion will usually be required (see below).

Width of the QRS complex

Measure the QRS complex to establish whether it is narrow or broad; this is particularly important when the child has a tachycardia (Biarent *et al.*, 2010):

- *QRS width less than 0.08 seconds (<2 small squares)* – this is a normal width, indicating that the tachycardia is either sinus tachycardia or SVT.
- *QRS width longer than 0.08 seconds (>2 small squares) or greater* – although in infants and children a broad complex tachyarrhythmia is more likely to be supraventricular than ventricular in origin (Benson *et al.*, 1982), when the child is decompensated, the tachyarrhythmia must be considered to be ventricular in origin unless it is proven to be supraventricular in origin (Biarent *et al.*, 2010).

Treatment of bradycardia, sinus tachycardia, SVT and VT is discussed below.

Treatment of sinus bradycardia and sinus tachycardia

Treatment of sinus bradycardia

- Follow the ABCDE approach.
- Deliver 100% oxygen, ideally using a non-rebreather mask. Provide effective ventilation if required.
- If the heart rate is less than 60 beats per minute and the child is poorly perfused, begin chest compressions and administer adrenaline 10 µg/kg intravenously (see Chapter 8).
- If the cause of the bradycardia is thought to be increased vagal tone, consider atropine 10 µg/kg (with a maximum of 600 µg) intravenously (Advanced Life Support Group, 2011).
- Although cardiac pacing is not usually helpful in this situation (Cummins *et al.*, 1993), consider it if there is atrioventricular block or sinus node dysfunction that has not responded to oxygenation, ventilation, chest compressions and other medications (Biarent *et al.*, 2010).

Treatment of sinus tachycardia

- Follow the ABCDE approach.
- Identify and treat (if necessary) the underlying cause.

Recognition and treatment of supraventricular tachycardia and ventricular tachycardia

Supraventricular tachycardia

SVT (see Fig. 6.9) is the most common non-arrest cardiac arrhythmia in children and the most common cardiac arrhythmia in infants that produces cardiovascular instability (Advanced Life Support Group, 2011). The ventricular rate in SVT is typically over 220 per minute, and the QRS complexes are narrow. Ideally, a 12-lead ECG should be recorded to help confirm the diagnosis.

Differentiating between sinus tachycardia and SVT

Differentiating between sinus tachycardia and SVT can sometimes be difficult. The Advanced Life Support Group (2011) suggests that the following characteristics will assist correct ECG interpretation:

- Sinus tachycardia if the *rate* is <200 per minute, SVT if it is >220 per minute
- Whether *P waves* can be identified: upright P waves in leads I and AVF suggest sinus tachycardia, and negative P waves in II, III and AVF suggest SVT
- *Rate and regularity* – these vary in sinus tachycardia and are constant in SVT
- *Onset and termination* – these are gradual in sinus tachycardia and abrupt in SVT
- A history of *shock* is usually present with sinus tachycardia

The child's age, ventricular rate, duration of SVT and ventricular function prior to the onset all influence the haemodynamic effect of SVT (American Academy of Pediatrics, 2000).

Treatment of supraventricular tachycardia

- Follow the *ABCDE approach*.
- *Vagal manoeuvres* – e.g. soaking a flannel or similar in iced cold water and placing it briefly over the child's face. Alternatively, if the child is cooperating, ask him or her to blow through a drinking straw or try to blow the plunger out of a syringe (Fig. 6.11). These manoeuvres can also be used in a child who is decompensated as long as they do not delay chemical or electrical cardioversion (Sreeram & Wren, 1990).
- *Chemical cardioversion* – adenosine 0.1 mg/kg (to a maximum of 6 mg) intravenously followed by flushing with 2–5 mL 0.9% saline. If this dose is ineffective, consider adenosine 0.2 mg/kg (to a maximum of 12 mg) intravenously followed by flushing with 2–5 mL 0.9% saline (Resuscitation Council (UK), 2011).
- *Electrical cardioversion* – this is the treatment of choice if the child is decompensated (particularly if he or she is unconscious) (see Chapter 7).

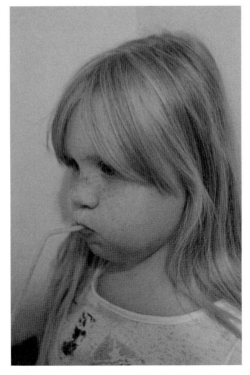

Fig. 6.11 Example of a vagal manoeuvre: blowing into a straw.

Ventricular tachycardia

VT (see Fig. 6.10), a rare cardiac arrhythmia in childhood, is characterised by a rapid QRS rate and broad (0.12 seconds or greater) QRS complexes. Causes include poisoning, hyperkalaemia and cardiac surgery. If possible, a 12-lead ECG should be recorded and analysed with the help of a paediatric cardiologist (Advanced Life Support Group, 2011). This will sometimes result in a loss of cardiac output, requiring urgent defibrillation (see Chapter 8).

Treatment of VT

- Follow the ABCDE approach.
- Seek expert help.

- Synchronised electrical cardioversion is the treatment of choice if the child is decompensated (particularly if he or she is unconscious) (see Chapter 7).
- If the child is pulseless, urgent defibrillation and CPR are required (see Chapter 7).

Summary

In this chapter, the conduction system of the heart together with the ECG and its relation to cardiac contraction have been described. A suggested ECG electrode placement for ECG monitoring has been outlined, together with the problems that can be encountered with ECG monitoring. The management of cardiac arrhythmias has been discussed. The principles of recognition and treatment of SVT and VT have been outlined.

References

Advanced Life Support Group (2011) *Advanced Paediatric Life Support*, 5th edn. Wiley Blackwell, Oxford.

American Academy of Pediatrics (2000) *Pediatric Education for Prehospital Professionals*. Jones & Bartlett, Sudbury, MA.

Benson, D, Jr., Smith, W., Dunnigan, A. *et al.* (1982) Mechanisms of regular wide QRS tachycardia in infants and children. *American Journal of Cardiology*, **49**, 1778–1788.

Biarent D, Bingham R, Christoph E *et al.* (2010) European Resuscitation Council Guidelines for Resuscitation Section 6. Paediatric life support (2010) *Resuscitation*, **81**, 1364–1388.

Cummins, R., Graves, J., Larsen, M. *et al.* (1993) Out-of-hospital transcutaneous pacing by emergency medical technicians in patients with asystolic cardiac arrest. *New England Journal of Medicine*, **328**, 1377–1382.

Jevon, P. (2009) *Advanced Cardiac Life Support*, 2nd edn. Wiley Blackwell, Oxford.

Resuscitation Council (UK) (2011) *Paediatric Immediate Life Support*, 2nd edn. Resuscitation Council (UK), London.

Sreeram, N. & Wren, C. (1990) Supraventricular tachycardia in infants: response to initial treatment. *Archives of Disease in Childhood*, **65**, 127–129.

Chapter 7

Defibrillation and Electrical Cardioversion

Introduction

Defibrillation can be defined as the passage of an electrical current through the myocardium of sufficient magnitude to depolarise a critical mass of myocardium, enabling coordinated electrical activity to resume and spontaneous circulation to return (Deakin *et al.*, 2010).

Although defibrillation is rare in the paediatric arrest situation, when it is indicated it is important to ensure that it is performed rapidly, safely and effectively. A knowledge of the principles of defibrillation is therefore required.

Synchronised electrical cardioversion is the timed delivery (to coincide with the R wave) of a defibrillatory shock and can be used to treat supraventicular tachycardia and ventricular tachy-cardia (VT) with a pulse (Resuscitation Council (UK), 2011).

The aim of this chapter is for the reader to understand the principles of defibrillation and electrical cardioversion.

Learning objectives

At the end of this chapter, the reader will be able to:

- Describe ventricular fibrillation (VF)
- Discuss the physiology of defibrillation
- Outline the factors affecting successful defibrillation
- Discuss the safety issues related to defibrillation

Paediatric Advanced Life Support: A Practical Guide for Nurses, Second Edition. Phil Jevon.
© 2012 Phil Jevon. Published 2012 by Blackwell Publishing Ltd.

- Describe the procedure for manual defibrillation
- Describe the procedure for automated external defibrillation
- Describe the procedure for emergency synchronised cardioversion
- Discuss the new technological advances in defibrillation

Ventricular fibrillation

> The cardiac pump is thrown out of gear, and the last of its vital energy is dissipated in a violent and prolonged turmoil of fruitless activity in the ventricular walls. (McWilliam, 1889)

In VF, the myocardium is depolarising at random, resulting in uncoordinated electrical activity, with a subsequent loss of cardiac output and cardiac arrest.

ECG characteristics

The ECG trace (see Fig. 1.3) is highly characteristic, with bizarre and chaotic waveforms. Initially, the amplitude and waveform in VF deteriorate rapidly, reflecting the depletion of myocardial high-energy phosphate stores (Jevon, 2009). If untreated, asystole will ensue.

Incidence

Compared with adults, VF in children is very rare, occurring in approximately 7–15% of paediatric and adolescent arrests (Mogayzel *et al.*, 1995; Atkins *et al.*, 2009).

Causes

A number of causes of VF in children have been reported, including trauma, congenital heart disease, long QT interval, drug overdose and hypothermia (Kuisma *et al.*, 1995; Hickey *et al.*, 1995; Sirbaugh *et al.*, 1999).

Treatment

Early defibrillation is the definitive treatment; the chances of success decline substantially (by approximately 10%) with each passing minute of delay in defibrillating (Resuscitation Council (UK), 2011; Waalewijn *et al.*, 2001). There is a slower decline if there is adequate basic life support (Jevon, 2009).

Pulseless ventricular tachycardia

Pulseless VT (see Fig. 1.3) is treated the same as VF. See Chapter 6 for a discussion of VT.

Mechanics of defibrillation

Critical mass of myocardium

The heart can respond to an extrinsic electrical impulse just as it can respond to an impulse from the sinoatrial node or from an ectopic focus. It is thought that successful defibrillation occurs when a critical mass of myocardium is depolarised by the passage of an electric current (Jevon, 2009). If a critical mass (75–90%) of the cells are in the same phase (recovery or repolarisation) when the current is removed, defibrillation occurs and the sinoatrial node or another intrinsic pacemaker can then regain control (Jevon, 2009).

Factors affecting success

Success will depend on the actual current flow rather than the energy of the shock. This flow of current is influenced by transthoracic impedance (the resistance of the chest tissues), the electrode position and the shock energy delivered. Only a small proportion of the energy delivered actually reaches the myocardium, so an effective technique is essential to optimise the chances of successful defibrillation.

Types of defibrillator

There are two types of defibrillator: automatic (automated external defibrillator, or AED) and manual. Some defibrillators, particularly those used in hospital, use a combination of both types.

Automated external defibrillators

AEDs are sophisticated, reliable, safe, computerised devices that deliver defibrillatory shocks when appropriate to persons in

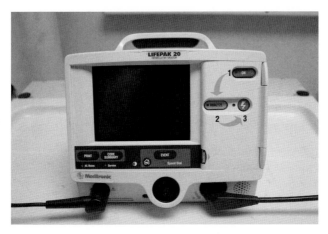

Fig. 7.1 Manual defibrillator with an automated (advisory) mode.

cardiopulmonary arrest (Resuscitation Council (UK), 2011). They are simple to use; voice and/or visual prompts provide guidance to the operator, enabling them to be easily used by both health-care professionals and lay persons. A few AEDs have an ECG display and a facility to enable the operator to switch from auto-mated to manual mode (Jevon, 2009). AEDs cannot be used for synchronised electrical cardioversion. The use of AEDs in chil-dren is discussed at length later in the chapter.

Manual defibrillators

Manual defibrillators require the operator to interpret the ECG and to select the appropriate level of shock energy. They are pre-ferred to an AED for use in a paediatric arrest because the appro-priate energy level specific for the child can be selected (Biarent *et al.*, 2010). Many manual defibrillators used in hospital also have an automated mode, i.e. similar to that of an AED (Fig. 7.1).

Monophasic and biphasic waveforms

There are basically two types of waveform: monophasic and biphasic (Deakin *et al.*, 2010):

- *Monophasic waveform* – the shock current flow is unipolar (i.e. flows in one direction). Monophasic defibrillators are no longer being manufactured but are still in use.

- *Biphasic waveform* – the shock current flow goes in one direction and is then reversed. This is superior to a monophasic waveform and features in all new defibrillators. Biphasic waveforms are at least as effective as monophasic waveforms, and certainly cause less harm to the myocardium.

Self-adhesive defibrillation pads or defibrillation paddles

Self-adhesive defibrillation pads
Self-adhesive defibrillation pads are used with AEDs and are usually now used with manual defibrillators. They enable hands-free defibrillation so that the person defibrillating can stand at a safe distance from the child/bed and chest compressions can continue while the defibrillator is charging. They are safer, more effective and preferable to the traditional defibrillation paddles. Some AEDs have paediatric attenuated devices, typically for use in children aged 1–8 years.

Defibrillation paddles
The traditional defibrillation paddles are now rarely used (Resuscitation Council (UK), 2011). If they are used, it is important to apply defibrillation gel pads to the chest.

Factors affecting successful defibrillation

As well as early defibrillation following the onset of VF (see above), there are a number of factors that can influence the likelihood of successful defibrillation. These will now be discussed.

Shock energy
Energy levels that are set too low will fail to defibrillate a critical mass of the myocardium, while those set too high may damage the myocardium and surrounding tissues. Selecting the appropriate energy levels reduces the number of repetitive shocks and limits myocardial damage (Biarent *et al.*, 2010).

The optimum shock energy for defibrillation in infants and children has yet to be determined (Biarent *et al.*, 2010). The Resuscitation Council (UK) (2011) recommends a shock energy dose of 4J/kg (biphasic or monophasic) up to a maximum of 360J for a monophasic defibrillator and 150–200J for a biphasic defibrillator for the first shock. Biphasic defibrillators have been shown to be more effective than monophasic ones.

Transthoracic impedance
If defibrillation is to be successful, sufficient electrical current needs to pass through the chest and depolarise a critical mass of myocardium. Transthoracic impedance is the resistance to the flow of current through the chest – the greater the resistance, the lower the current flow. Several factors can influence transthoracic impedance, and correct defibrillation technique is essential to minimise their negative effects and maximise flow of current to the myocardium.

Position of self-adhesive defibrillation pads and paddles
The self-adhesive defibrillation pads or paddles should be placed to maximise the current flow through the myocardium. The polarity is unimportant for defibrillation (Resuscitation Council (UK), 2011). The most commonly used position is one paddle on the anterior chest, just to the right of the sternum (not over the sternum) below the right clavicle, and the other in the mid-axillary line on the left side of the chest (Resuscitation Council (UK), 2011).

The anteroposterior paddle position, although theoretically superior, is not practical in the emergency situation. However, it may be required if an infant requires defibrillation and only adult-sized self-adhesive defibrillation pads or paddles are available. This position may also be considered in a child with an implantable cardioverter-defibrillator (ICD) and/or pacemaker: the pads will need to be at least 12 cm away from the ICD/pacemaker site (Resuscitation Council (UK), 2011).

Size of self-adhesive defibrillation pads and defibrillation paddles
The larger the size of the pad, the lower the transthoracic impedance. The general recommendation is to use the largest size paddles or defibrillation pads that fit on the infant or child's chest in the anterolateral or anteroposterior position without them touching each other (Tibballs *et al.*, 2010).

For self-adhesive defibrillation pads, manufacturers usually recommend the large 'adult pads' for children over 8 years of age, and the small paediatric pads for those under 8. What is important, however, is that the pads do not touch. If paediatric pads are not available, adult pads can be used (see later).

If using defibrillation paddles, use paddles that are (Biarent *et al.*, 2010):

- 4.5 cm in diameter for infants and children weighing less than 10 kg (Fig. 7.2)
- 8–12 cm in diameter for children heavier than 10 kg (older than 1 year) (Fig. 7.3)

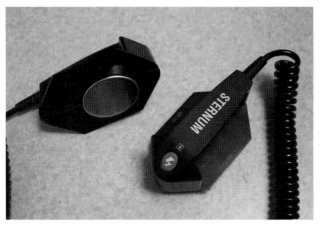

Fig. 7.2 4.5 cm diameter defibrillation paddles for infants and children weighing less than 10 kg.

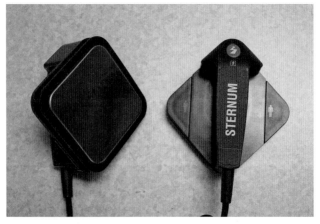

Fig. 7.3 8–12 cm diameter defibrillation paddles for children weighing more than 10 kg (older than 1 year).

If paediatric paddles are not available and defibrillation is required in an infant, adult paddles can be used, but they should be positioned in the anteroposterior position (Advanced Life Support Group, 2011).

Interface between self-adhesive defibrillation pads and the child's skin
If the child's skin is very clammy, drying the chest before applying the self-adhesive pads will help to improve contact. It is also important to 'smooth down' the pads to help ensure good skin contact.

Interface between the paddles and the child's skin
If using paddles, defibrillation gel pads should be used with defibrillation paddles to reduce the impedance between the paddles and the skin. (They also can help to prevent skin burns.)

Paddle pressure
If using defibrillation paddles, press them down firmly on the chest wall to help ensure good contact and reduce transthoracic impedance (Biarent *et al.*, 2010).

Safety issues and defibrillation

Confirmation of cardiac arrest

It is important to confirm cardiac arrest and ascertain that the ECG trace is displaying a shockable rhythm requiring defibrillation. It is important to reconfirm that the child is still in a shockable rhythm before defibrillating.

Minimising the risk of skin burns

If using defibrillation paddles, ensure that defibrillation gel pads have been applied to the child's bare chest to minimise the risk of skin burns (as well as improve conduction).

Minimising the risk of bystanders receiving a shock

Avoid direct and indirect contact with the child (Gibbs *et al.*, 1990). All personnel should stand well away from the bed and not touch the child or anything attached to the patient or bed, such as intravenous infusions or their stands. Be wary of wet surroundings. Shout 'Stand clear!', and ensure that everyone is clear before defibrillating the child.

Minimising the risk of a fire

There have been case reports describing how sparks from incorrectly applied defibrillator paddles have, in an oxygen-enriched atmosphere, caused a fire (Ward, 1996); one such case occurred at a paediatric arrest (Theodorou *et al.* 2003). There are no such reports concerning the use of defibrillation pads (Deakin *et al.*, 2010).

To minimise the risk of a fire during attempted defibrillation, the following precautions are recommended (Deakin *et al.*, 2010; Resuscitation Council (UK), 2011):

- Remove any oxygen delivery device, e.g. oxygen mask, bag-valve-mask device or nasal cannula, to at least 1 m away from the child's chest.
- If the bag-valve device is attached to the tracheal tube or supraglottic airway device, it is safe to leave it attached.
- If the child is connected to a ventilator, it is safe to leave the ventilator tubing (breathing circuit) attached to the tracheal tube.
- If using defibrillation paddles, apply firm pressure to minimise the risk of sparks.

Procedure for manual defibrillation

Resuscitation Guidelines 2010

The Resuscitation Guidelines 2010 relating to defibrillation stress the importance of (Deakin *et al.*, 2010):

- Early, uninterrupted chest compressions
- Minimising the duration of the pre-defibrillation and post-defibrillation pauses
- Continuing chest compressions while the defibrillator is charging up
- Resuming chest compressions immediately following defibrillation

- Limiting the interruption for chest compression to no longer than 5 seconds
- Performing a very quick safety check to limit the pre-defibrillation pause to chest compressions
- Considering using up to three-stacked defibrillation shocks if VF/VT occurs in the paediatric catheter laboratory, in the early postoperative period following cardiac surgery or in a witnessed VF/VT cardiac arrest when the child is already connected to a manual defibrillator.

Using a manual defibrillator is preferred to using an AED in a paediatric arrest because the required number of joules can be selected (Biarent *et al.*, 2010).

Procedure for manual defibrillation using self-adhesive pads

1. Confirm cardiac arrest, ensure that the paediatric cardiac arrest team has been alerted, and request the defibrillator and cardiac arrest trolley.
2. Provide initial five ventilations followed by cardiopulmonary resuscitation (CPR), 15 compressions to 2 ventilations.
3. As soon as the defibrillator arrives, switch it on. Ensure that CPR continues.
4. Apply self-adhesive defibrillation pads to the child's bare chest following the manufacturer's recommendations (check the pictures on the pads). This will usually be the anterolateral position (Fig. 7.4), although in an infant, the anteroposterior position will probably be used. Ensure that CPR continues.
5. Plan actions before requesting that CPR is stopped for ECG interpretation to take place – these actions need to be communicated to the team.
6. Once the pads are in place and connected to the defibrillator, ask the team to stop CPR and analyse the ECG trace.
7. If a shockable rhythm is identified, request that chest compressions are restarted, select the appropriate shock energy (4 J/kg), and charge up the defibrillator.
8. Once the defibrillator is charged, ask the person performing chest compressions and other colleagues to stand clear, and if necessary remove any oxygen delivery device (see above). Once everyone is clear, confirm that the child is still in a shockable rhythm.

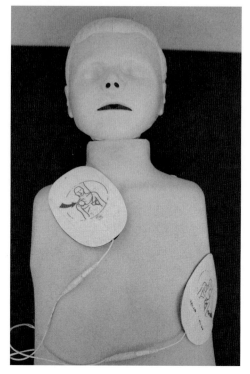

Fig. 7.4 Placement of self-adhesive defibrillation pads.

9. Defibrillate the child by pressing the shock button(s).
10. Immediately recommence CPR, 15 compressions to 2 ventilations, for a further 2 minutes, during which time the cardiac arrest team leader will prepare the team for the next pause in CPR.
11. After 2 minutes, repeat steps 5–9 as appropriate

Points to note

• In a witnessed arrest, where a the child is already attached to a defibrillator monitor that displays VF, immediate defibrillation will usually take priority over initial ventilation.
• Up to three shocks may be given at a time on rare occasions (see above). Wearing gloves may provide some protection against accidental shock.

Procedure for automated external defibrillation

Use of automated external defibrillation in children

Case reports have shown that AEDs can be used safely and successfully in children older than 1 year of age (Gurnett & Atkins, 2000; Konig *et al.*, 2005). They can accurately interpret cardiac arrhythmias in children and are very unlikely to advise a shock inappropriately (Cecchin *et al.*, 2001; Atkinson *et al.*, 2003; Atkins *et al.*, 2008). The use of AEDs is therefore recommended in all children over 1 year of age (Samson *et al.*, 2003).

Most manufacturers now supply paediatric pads or software, which typically attenuate the output of the AED to 50–75J (Jorgenson *et al.*, 2002) and are recommended for children between 1 and 8 years of age (Tang *et al.*, 2002; Berg *et al.*, 2004). However, if an AED with attenuated shock or a manually adjustable defibrillator is not available, an unmodified adult AED can be used in children over 1 year of age (Berg *et al.*, 2005). If it is possible that an AED may need to be used in a paediatric arrest, it is important to check that the AED has been tested against paediatric arrhythmias (Biarent *et al.*, 2010).

In infants, shockable rhythms are extremely rare unless there is underlying cardiac disease (Rodriguez-Nunez *et al.*, 2006; Samson *et al.*, 2006; Atkins *et al.*, 2009). The only evidence to support the use of an AED in infants (<1 year of age) comes from case reports (Bar-Cohen *et al.*, 2005; Divekar & Soni, 2006). Where there is a history of cardiac disease, the risk:benefit ratio may be favourable, and the use of an AED, ideally with a dose attenuator, should be considered (Biarent *et al.*, 2010).

Procedure

1. Confirm cardiac arrest, ensure that the paediatric cardiac arrest team has been alerted, and request the AED and cardiac arrest trolley.
2. Provide initial five ventilations followed by CPR, 15 compressions to 2 ventilations.
3. Switch on the AED. If appropriate, and if available, connect a paediatric attenuated device. Ensure that CPR continues.
4. Follow spoken and/or visual prompts. Ensure that CPR continues.

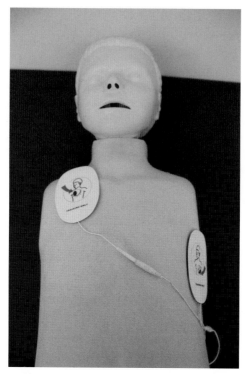

Fig. 7.5 Placement of automated external defibrillator pads in a child.

5. Ensure the child's chest is exposed, and dry the chest. Ensure that CPR continues.
6. Apply self-adhesive defibrillation pads to the child's bare chest following the manufacturer's recommendations (check the pictures on the pads) (Fig. 7.5). This will usually be the anterolateral position, although in an infant, the anteroposterior position will probably be used). Ensure that CPR continues.
7. Stand clear while the AED performs an ECG analysis, and ensure nobody touches the child during the ECG analysis; this is to prevent artefactual errors during the analysis (Sedgwick *et al.*, 1992). In addition, movement of the child can interrupt and delay it.
8. If shock is advised, shout 'Stand clear!' and perform a visual check to ensure all staff are clear; if necessary, request that

any oxygen delivery device is move to at least 1 m away from the child. The AED will automatically charge up to a predefined energy level, typically 50–70 J.

9. Defibrillate the child by pressing the shock button.
10. Immediately recommence CPR following the AED's instructions, 15 compressions to 2 ventilations. The AED will usually carry out a reanalysis after 2 minutes.

Procedure for synchronised electrical cardioversion

Indications

Synchronised cardioversion is a reliable method of converting a tachyarrhythmia, e.g. a supraventricular tachycardia or VT with a pulse, to sinus rhythm (Resuscitation Council (UK), 2011). Due to the associated risks, it is generally only undertaken when chemical intervention has been unsuccessful and/or if the child is decompensated (haemodynamically compromised).

Synchronisation mode

The shock should be delivered on the R wave and not on the vulnerable T wave; synchronising the delivered energy with the ECG will reduce the risk of inducing VF (Lown, 1967). This is accomplished by securing a reliable ECG trace (usually in lead II) using the defibrillator monitor and by pressing the 'sync' button on the defibrillator. A dot or arrow should only appear on the R waves.

Procedure

> If the child is not unconscious, sedation or anaesthesia will be required – seek expert help.

1. Attach the ECG leads and establish an accurate ECG trace. Lead II is usually selected. The defibrillator should be used for cardiac monitoring, otherwise synchronisation will not be possible
2. Activate the 'sync' button on the defibrillator.

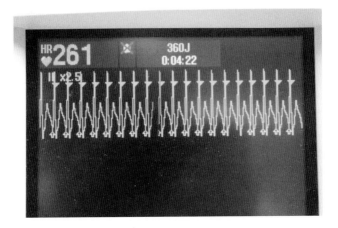

Fig. 7.6 Synchronisation on the R waves.

3. Check that only the R waves are being synchronised; a dot or an arrow should appear on each R wave and not on other parts of the ECG complex (e.g. tall T waves) (Fig. 7.6). It may be necessary to alter the ECG gain to increase the size of the R waves so that reliable synchronisation can take place.

4. Apply the self-adhesive defibrillation pads as advised by the manufacturer.

5. Select the required energy dose – 0.5–1 J/kg (which is increased to 2 J/kg for subsequent shocks; Advanced Life Support Group, 2011).

6. Press the charge button on the paddles to charge the defibrillator and shout 'Stand clear!

7. Perform a visual check of the area to ensure that all personnel are clear.

8. Check the monitor to ensure that the child is still in the tachyarrhythmia that requires synchronised electrical cardioversion. Also check that the synchronised button is still activated and is synchronising on just the R waves.

9. Press the shock button(s) to discharge the shock. There will be a slight delay (until the next R wave) between pressing the shock button(s) and shock discharge.

10. Check the ECG monitor.

11. Repeat the procedure if necessary.

Points to note

- If possible, consent should be obtained from the child or the parents/carers.
- CPR equipment should be immediately available in case of cardiac arrest following the procedure.
- Following cardioversion, the 'sync' button will usually need to be reactivated if further cardioversion is required. However, on some defibrillators, the 'sync' button will remain activated once pressed and therefore needs to be switched off once no further cardioversion is required.
- Antiarrhythmic therapy, e.g. amiodarone, may be required

Summary

The ECG characteristics and pathophysiology of VF have been described. The factors affecting successful defibrillation, together with safety issues, have been discussed. The procedures for manual defibrillation, automated external defibrillation and emergency synchronised cardioversion have been described. If indicated, defibrillation should be performed rapidly, safely and effectively.

References

Advanced Life Support Group (2011) *Advanced Paediatric Life Support*, 5th edn. Wiley Blackwell, Oxford.

Atkins, D., Scott, W., Blaufox, A., *et al.* (2008) Sensitivity and specificity of an automated external defibrillator algorithm designed for pediatric patients. *Resuscitation*, **76**, 168–174.

Atkins, D., Everson-Stewart, S., Sears, G.K., *et al.* (2009) Epidemiology and outcomes from out-of-hospital cardiac arrest in children: the Resuscitation Outcomes Consortium Epistry–Cardiac Arrest. *Circulation*, **119**, 1484–1491.

Atkinson, E., Mikysa, B., Conway, J.A., *et al.* (2003) Specificity and sensitivity of automated external defibrillator rhythm analysis in infants and children. *Annals of Emergency Medicine*, **42**, 185–196.

Bar-Cohen, Y., Walsh, E., Love, B. & Cecchin, F. (2005) First appropriate use of automated external defibrillator in an infant. *Resuscitation*, **67**, 135–137.

Berg, R., Chapman, F., Berg, M., *et al.* (2004) Attenuated adult biphasic shocks compared with weight-based monophasic shocks in a swine model of prolonged pediatric ventricular fibrillation. *Resuscitation*, **61**, 189–197.

Berg, R., Samson, R., Berg, M., *et al.* (2005) Better outcome after pediatric defibrillation dosage than adult dosage in a swine model of pediatric ventricular fibrillation. *Journal of the American College of Cardiology*, **45**, 786–789.

Biarent, D., Bingham, R., Christoph, E., *et al.* (2010) European Resuscitation Council Guidelines for Resuscitation Section 6. Paediatric life support (2010). *Resuscitation*, **81**, 1364–1388.

Cecchin, F., Jorgenson, D.B., Berul, C.I., *et al.* (2001) Is arrhythmia detection by automatic external defibrillator accurate for children? Sensitivity and specificity of an automatic external defibrillator algorithm in 696 pediatric arrhythmias. *Circulation*, **103**, 2483–2488.

Deakin, C., Nolan, J., Sunde, K. & Kosterd, R. (2010) European Resuscitation Council Guidelines for Resuscitation 2010 Section 3. Electrical therapies: automated external defibrillators, defibrillation, cardioversion and pacing. *Resuscitation*, **81**, 1293–1304.

Divekar, A. & Soni, R. (2006) Successful parental use of an automated external defibrillator for an infant with long-QT syndrome. *Pediatrics*, **118**, e526–e529.

Gibbs, W., Eisenberg, M. & Damon, S. (1990) Dangers of defibrillation: injuries to personnel during patient resuscitation. *American Journal of Emergency Medicine*, **8**, 101–104.

Gurnett, C. & Atkins, D. (2000) Successful use of a biphasic waveform automated external defibrillator in a high-risk child. *American Journal of Cardiology*, **8**, 1051–1053.

Hickey, R., Cohen, D., Strausbaugh, S. & Dietrich, A. (1995) Pediatric patients requiring CPR in the prehospital setting. *Annals of Emergency Medicine*, **25**, 495–501.

Jevon, P. (2009) *Advanced Cardiac Life Support*, 2nd edn. Wiley Blackwell, London.

Jorgenson, D., Morgan, C., Snyder, D., *et al.* (2002. Energy attenuator for pediatric application of an automated external defibrillator. *Critical Care Medicine*, **30**, S145–S147.

Konig, B., Benger, J. & Goldsworthy, L. (2005) Automatic external defibrillation in a 6 year old. *Archives of Disease in Childhood*, **90**, 310–311.

Kuisma, M., Suominen, P. & Korpela, R. (1995) Paediatric out-of-hospital cardiac arrests: epidemiology and outcome. *Resuscitation*, **30**, 141–150.

Lown, B. (1967) Electrical reversion of cardiac arrhythmias. *British Heart Journal*, **29**, 469–489.

McWilliam, J. (1889) Electrical stimulation of the heart in man. *BMJ*, **1**, 348–350.

Mogayzel, C., Quan, L., Graves, J., *et al.* (1995) Out -of- hospital ventricular fibrillation in children and adolescents: causes and outcomes. *Annals of Emergency Medicine*, **25**, 484–491.

Resuscitation Council (UK) (2011) *Paediatric Immediate Life Support*, 2nd edn. Resuscitation Council (UK), London.

Rodriguez-Nunez, A., Lopez-Herce, J., Garcia, C., *et al.* (2006) Pediatric defibrillation after cardiac arrest: initial response and outcome. *Critical Care*, **10**, R113.

Samson, R., Berg, R. & Bingham, R. (2003) Pediatric Advanced Life Support Task Force ILCoR. Use of automated external defibrillators for children: an update. An advisory statement from the Pediatric Advanced Life Support Task Force, International Liaison Committee on Resuscitation. *Resuscitation*, **57**, 237–243.

Samson, R., Nadkarni, V., Meaney, P., *et al.* (2006) Outcomes of in-hospital ventricular fibrillation in children. *New England Journal of Medicine*, **354**, 2328–2339.

Sedgwick, M.L., Watson, J., Dalziel, K., *et al.* (1992) Efficacy of out of hospital defibrillation by ambulance technicians using automated external defibrillators: the Heartstart Scotland Project. *Resuscitation*, **24**, 73–87.

Sirbaugh, P., Pepe, P., Shook, J., *et al.* (1999) A prospective, population-based study of the demographics, epidemiology, management, and outcome of out-of-hospital pediatric cardiopulmonary arrest. *Annals of Emergency Medicine*, **33**, 174–184.

Tang, W., Weil, M., Jorgenson, D., *et al.* (2002) Fixed-energy biphasic waveform defibrillation in a pediatric model of cardiac arrest and resuscitation. *Critical Care Medicine*, **30**, 2736–2741.

Theodorou, A., Gutierrez, J. & Berg, R. (2003) Fire attributable to a defibrillation attempt in a neonate. *Pediatrics*, **112**, 677–679.

Tibballs, J., Carter, B., Kiraly, N., *et al.* (2010) Biphasic DC shock cardioverting doses for paediatric atrial dysrhythmias. *Resuscitation*, **81**, 1101–1104.

Waalewijn, R., de Vos, R., Tijssen, J. & Koster, R. (2001) Survival models for out-of-hospital cardiopulmonary resuscitation from the perspectives of the bystander, the first responder, and the paramedic. *Resuscitation*, **51**, 113–122.

Ward, M. (1996) Risk of fires when using defibrillators in an oxygen enriched atmosphere. *Resuscitation*, **31**, 173.

Chapter 8

Paediatric Advanced Life Support

Introduction

Paediatric advanced life support (PALS) is the term used to describe the more specialised techniques employed to support breathing and circulation during paediatric cardiopulmonary resuscitation (CPR), as well as specific treatment used to try and restore cardiac output.

The Resuscitation Council (UK) Paediatric Advanced Life Support algorithm (2011) (Fig. 8.1) is universally applicable, although specific modifications are required to maximise the likelihood of success in some special situations (see Chapters 9 and 10).

The aim of this chapter is for the reader to understand the principles of PALS.

Learning objectives

At the end of this chapter, the reader will be able to:

- Outline the Resuscitation Council's PALS algorithm
- Outline the principles of intraosseous infusion
- Discuss the tracheal route for drug administration
- Discuss the use of resuscitation drugs
- Discuss the treatment of potential reversible causes of paediatric cardiac arrest
- Outline the treatment of bradyarrhythmias and tachyarrhythmias

Paediatric Advanced Life Support: A Practical Guide for Nurses, Second Edition.
Phil Jevon.
© 2012 Phil Jevon. Published 2012 by Blackwell Publishing Ltd.

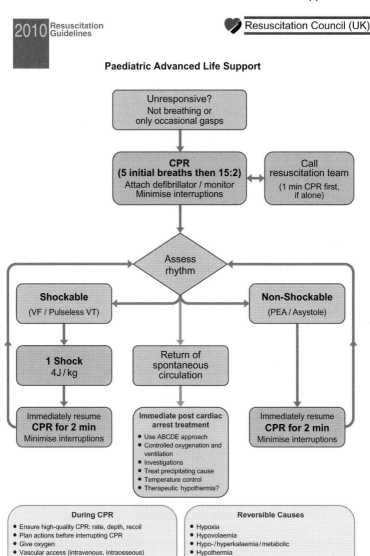

Fig. 8.1 Resuscitation Council (UK) Paediatric Advanced Life Support algorithm (2011), reproduced with kind permission. CPR, cardiopulmonary resuscitation; PEA, pulseless electrical activity; VT, ventricular tachycardia.

Resuscitation Council (UK) PALS algorithm

The Resuscitation Council (UK) PALS algorithm (Fig. 8.1) is designed to be an aide-mémoire, reminding the practitioner of the important aspects of assessment and treatment for a paediatric cardiac arrest. It is not designed to be comprehensive or limiting. Each step that follows in the algorithm assumes that the previous one has been unsuccessful. Looping the algorithm reinforces the concept of constant assessment and reassessment.

Cardiopulmonary resuscitation (five initial breaths – the 15:2)

PALS initially involves the establishment of effective basic life support and ventilation. The airway should be opened, and positive-pressure ventilation with a high inspired oxygen concentration should be provided. In some situations, these interventions may be all that is required to resuscitate the child.

While CPR is started, a colleague should call the resuscitation team. In the unlikely event of a practitioner being alone, CPR should be performed for 1 minute first before the resuscitation team is called (Resuscitation Council (UK), 2011).

Call the resuscitation team (1 minute CPR first if alone)

Most hospitals should alert the resuscitation team by dialling 2222.

Attach the defibrillator/monitor

As soon as the defibrillator/monitor arrives, establish ECG monitoring. This will usually be with either self-adhesive defibrillation pads or standard ECG electrodes.

Self-adhesive defibrillation pads
If self-adhesive defibrillation pads are used, apply them following the manufacturer's recommendations. This is usually one pad to the right of the sternum below the clavicle, and one on the left side of the chest in the mid-axillary line (Fig. 8.2).

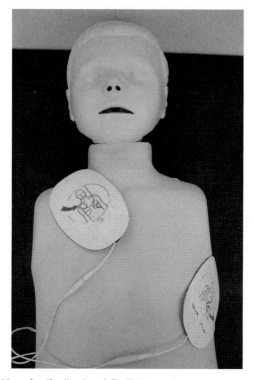

Fig. 8.2 Position of self-adhesive defibrillation pads.

Three-lead ECG monitoring

If three-lead ECG monitoring is used, select lead II on the ECG monitor and attach the ECG leads as follows (Fig. 8.3):

- *Red* on the right shoulder
- *Yellow* on the left shoulder
- *Green* on the left upper abdominal wall

Minimise interruptions

The importance of providing quality CPR and minimising interruptions to CPR has been discussed in Chapter 4. Throughout the resuscitation event, attempts should be made to minimise interruptions to CPR and chest compressions in particular. For example:

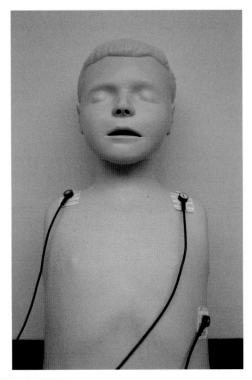

Fig. 8.3 Position for ECG electrodes.

- Plan proposed actions with the team before interrupting CPR
- Continue CPR while charging up the defibrillator
- Once the airway is secured, e.g. with a tracheal tube, provide asynchronous CPR, i.e. continuous chest compressions without pauses for ventilations
- Ideally, change the practitioner performing chest compressions when CPR has stopped for ECG rhythm assessment

Assess the rhythm

Ask the team to briefly stop CPR and assess the ECG rhythm. The presenting cardiac arrest arrhythmia can then be classified into one of two groups – shockable or non-shockable – depending on whether defibrillation is required. The appropriate pathway in the algorithm can then be followed. In a paediatric arrest, the ECG rhythm will most likely be a non-shockable rhythm.

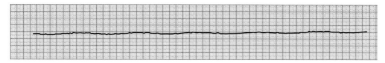

Fig. 8.4 Asystole.

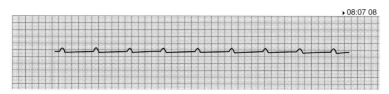

Fig. 8.5 P wave asystole.

Non-shockable (pulseless electrical activity/asystole)

If a non-shockable rhythm is identified, defibrillation is not indicated at this stage, and the non-shockable pathway of the algorithm should be followed. The two main non-shockable cardiac rhythms are asystole and pulseless electrical activity (PEA).

Asystole
Asystole (Fig. 8.4) is the most common cardiac arrest arrhythmia in children (Advanced Life Support Group, 2011). P waves may sometimes be seen (P wave asystole; Fig. 8.5). Care should be taken to ensure that the ECG trace is accurate and that the 'straight line' is not the result of a mechanical problem. Check that:

- The ECG leads or self-adhesive defibrillation pads have been correctly attached
- The correct monitoring lead has been selected (normally *lead II* if ECG electrodes are being used and *paddles* if self-adhesive defibrillation pads are being used)
- The ECG gain (ECG size) is not turned down low

Asystole is rarely a straight line. Spurious asystole may be displayed following defibrillation if monitoring is carried out through defibrillation paddles – the ECG trace should be confirmed by monitoring through the ECG leads. Cardiac pacing is ineffective in the management of asystole (Quan *et al.*, 1992).

Pulseless electrical activity

PEA is a clinical condition of cardiac arrest but in the presence of a normal or near-normal ECG trace. It can be either primary or secondary. Primary PEA results from failure of the myocardium to respond to electrical stimulation, e.g. in hypoxia; secondary PEA occurs when mechanical barriers to ventricular filling or cardiac output are present, e.g. tension pneumothorax. The child's optimal chance for survival rests with the prompt identification and treatment of any underlying cause (see below).

Non-shockable rhythm – immediately resume CPR for 2 minutes

Having confirmed a non-shockable rhythm, restart CPR immediately with 15 chest compressions to 2 ventilations for 2 minutes before reassessing the ECG rhythm. During this period of CPR (Biarent *et al.*, 2010; Resuscitation Council (UK), 2011):

- Ensure high-quality CPR – depth, rate and recoil
- Plan actions before interrupting CPR
- Deliver a high concentration of oxygen; e.g. continue with 15 L per minute attached to a bag-valve device
- Consider advanced airway intervention, e.g. tracheal intubation, and capnography
- Secure vascular access (intravenous, intraosseous)
- Administer adrenaline 10 µg/kg every 3–5 minutes
- Provide continuous chest compressions once an advanced airway, e.g. a tracheal tube, is in place
- Identify and correct reversible causes (see below)

Each loop of the algorithm provides a further opportunity, if one has not already occurred, to secure venous access and attempt tracheal intubation. The accuracy of the ECG trace should be regularly verified. Adrenaline is administered every 3–5 minutes. Sodium bicarbonate should be considered in a prolonged arrest and in an arrest associated with severe metabolic acidosis.

Shockable (ventricular fibrillation/pulseless ventricular tachycardia)

If ventricular fibrillation (VF) or pulseless ventricular tachycardia (VT) is identified (rare) (Fig. 1.3), defibrillation should be performed as soon as possible. The recommended energy for defibrillation is 4 J/kg regardless of whether the defibrillator is monophasic or biphasic. The principles of defibrillation were discussed in detail in chapter 7.

Shockable rhythm – immediately resume CPR for 2 minutes

Following defibrillation, restart CPR immediately with 15 chest compressions to 2 ventilations for 2 minutes before reassessing the ECG rhythm. During this period of CPR (Biarent *et al.*, 2010; Resuscitation Council (UK), 2011):

- Ensure high-quality CPR – depth, rate and recoil
- Plan actions before interrupting CPR
- Deliver a high concentration of oxygen; e.g. continue with 15 L per minute attached to a bag-valve device
- Consider advanced airway intervention, e.g. tracheal intubation, and capnography
- Secure vascular access (intravenous, intraosseous)
- After the third shock, administer adrenaline 10 μg/kg every 3–5 minutes
- Provide continuous chest compressions once an advanced airway, e.g. a tracheal tube, is in place
- Identify and correct reversible causes (see below)

Each loop of the algorithm provides a further opportunity, if one has not already occurred, to secure venous access and attempt tracheal intubation. The accuracy of the ECG trace should be regularly verified. Adrenaline is administered every 3–5 minutes.

In refractory VF (after the third shock), amiodarone 5 mg/kg should be administered and repeated after the fifth shock if necessary. Sodium bicarbonate should be considered in a prolonged arrest and in an arrest associated with severe metabolic acidosis.

Intraosseous infusion

Establishing vascular access is crucial for drug and fluid administration. However, obtaining intravenous access in a paediatric arrest can be very difficult, and any delay in securing it may compromise the resuscitation attempt. The intraosseous route is the emergency circulatory route of choice in paediatric resuscitation (Resuscitation Council (UK), 2011).

Intraosseous access is a quick, reliable and relatively easy method of establishing vascular access. It can be used for the administration of drugs, fluids and blood products in infants and small children in the resuscitation situation (Berg, 1984; Glaeser & Losek, 1986; McNamara *et al.*, 1987).

Advantages of intraosseus infusion

The advantages of intraosseous infusion include the following:

- It is quick to establish. In the majority of cases, it can be achieved within 30–60 seconds, even by practitioners with limited experience (Glaeser *et al.*, 1988).
- The onset of action and drug levels are comparable with those achieved by conventional intravenous access (Andropoulos *et al.*, 1990).
- Blood sampling for laboratory studies is possible (see below).

Bone marrow samples

Bone marrow samples can be taken for a number of tests including:

- Crossmatch for blood type or group (Brickman *et al.*, 1992)
- Chemical analysis (Johnson *et al.*, 1999; Ummenhofer *et al.*, 1994)
- Blood gas measurement – as long as no medication has been injected into the bone marrow cavity, blood gas values are comparable with central venous blood gas levels (Abdelmoneim *et al.*, 1999; Voelckel *et al.*, 2000)

As bone marrow samples can damage autoanalysers, they should preferably be assessed in a cartridge analyser (Biarent et al., 2010).

Sites for intraosseus infusion

The Resuscitation Council (UK) (2011) recommends the following sites for intraosseus infusion specifically to avoid the growth plates in the bones:

- The anteromedial surface of the tibia 2–3 cm below the tibial tuberosity – this is the most commonly used site for intraosseus infusion (Advanced Life Support Group, 2011). There is a large bone marrow cavity here and minimal risk to adjacent tissues
- The lower end of the tibia about 3 cm above the medial malleolus
- The lateral aspect of the distal femur about 3 cm above the lateral condyle

Intraosseus needles

Intraosseous needles are available in different sizes. The Resuscitation Council (UK) (2011) recommends:

- <6 months of age – size 18 gauge
- 6–18 months – size 16 gauge
- >18 months – size 14 gauge

Procedure for manual insertion of an intraosseus needle

1. Locate the site of access (see above).
2. Clean the site with antiseptic solution (if circumstances permit).
3. Select a size of intraosseus needle appropriate for the child's age (see above).
4. Check that the bevels of the outer needle and the internal stylet of the intraosseous needle are properly aligned.
5. Stabilise the child's leg. Using the palm of the non-dominant hand, grasp the thigh and knee above and lateral to the insertion site, and wrap the thumb and fingers around the knee. It is important to ensure that no part of your hand is allowed to rest behind the insertion site (under the leg).
6. Insert the needle into the bone at right angles to the long axis of the bone, in a slight caudal direction to avoid the epiphyseal plate. Adopt a gentle but firm twisting or drilling

technique. As it passes through the bony cortex into the marrow, a sudden drop in resistance should be felt. If the needle is in the correct position:
   – It should stay upright without support
   – It should be possible to aspirate bone marrow
   – Fluid can be injected through the needle, without evidence of its infiltrating the surrounding tissues.
7. Once successful insertion has been confirmed, flush the cannula, secure it with tape, and connect a primed infusion tubing with a three-way tap.
8. Send a bone marrow sample for laboratory studies (informing the technician that it is bone marrow to avoid unnecessary damage to laboratory equipment).
9. Use a 20 mL syringe to inject fluids and medications (Advanced Life Support Group, 2011). This is necessary to overcome resistance.
10. Flush with normal saline to ensure that the medications are delivered to the central circulation.

(Source: Advanced Life Support Group, 2011)

Complications of intraosseus infusion

Complications of intraosseous infusion do not often occur (Heinild *et al.*, 1974; Rosetti *et al.*, 1985), and the long-term effects of intraosseous infusion on the bone marrow and bone growth are minimal. However, the following complications have been reported:

• Fractured tibia (La Fleche *et al.*, 1989)
• Lower extremity compartment syndrome (Vidal *et al.*, 1993)
• Severe extravasation of medications (Simmons *et al.*, 1994)
• Osteomyelitis (Rosovsky *et al.*, 1994)

Although complications are rare, they can be severe. Consequently, intraosseous infusion should only be undertaken in critically ill infants and children (as a temporary measure until other venous access sites have been secured) (Fuchs *et al.*, 1991).

Semi-automated intraosseus devices

Several different intraosseus 'guns' or 'drills' are commercially available. They enable the rapid insertion of an intraosseous needle, using the same landmarks that are used in manual inser-

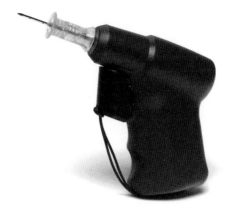

Fig. 8.6 EZ-IO device for intraosseous infusion.

tion (see above); however, the technique is less painful for the conscious child due to its rapidity of use (Advanced Life Support Group, 2011). One such device is the the EZ-IO drill (Shavano Park, TX, USA; Fig. 8.6) which uses three sizes of needle (Fig. 8.7).

The procedure for insertion of an intraosseus needle using the EZ-IO drill is as follows (Advanced Life Support Group, 2011):

1. Locate the site of access (see above).
2. Clean the site with antiseptic solution (if circumstances permit).
3. Select size of intraosseus needle appropriate for the child (see Fig. 8.7) and attach it to the drill (via the magnetic attachment).
4. Stabilise the child's leg. Using the palm of the non-dominant hand, grasp the thigh and knee above and lateral to the insertion site, and wrap the thumb and fingers around the knee. It is important to ensure that no part of your hand is allowed to rest behind the insertion site (under the leg).
5. Hold the drill and needle at 90 degrees to the skin surface.
6. Piece the skin with the needle (Fig. 8.8) without drilling, until bone is felt.
7. Press the drill button, drill and push continuously until there is a loss of resistance – there is a palpable 'give' as the needle breaches the cortex.

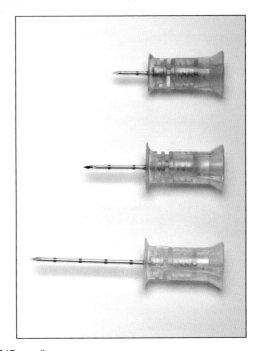

Fig. 8.7 EZ-IO needles.

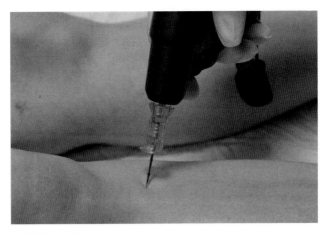

Fig. 8.8 EZ-IO drill obtaining intraosseous access.

8. Remove the drill, unscrew the trocar and confirm correct placement (by aspirating bone marrow, etc. – see above).
9. Once successful insertion has been confirmed, flush the cannula, secure it with tape, and connect a primed infusion tubing with a three-way tap.
10. Aspirate and discard 2 mL of aspirate before obtaining a bone marrow sample for laboratory studies (informing the technician that it is bone marrow to avoid unnecessary damage to laboratory equipment).
11. Use a 20 mL syringe to inject fluids and medications (Advanced Life Support Group, 2001). This is necessary to overcome resistance.
12. Flush with normal saline to ensure that medications are delivered to the central circulation.

Processing samples from an intraosseus aspiration using the EZ-IO product system has not been found to damage laboratory equipment. By alerting the laboratory or pathologist that the sample is from an intraosseus biopsy, they will be prepared to potentially observe stem cells and progenitor cells from the medullary space.

The intraosseous space is occupied by bone marrow that is held in place by a thick fibrin network. To obtain maximum flow rates, this thick fibrin mesh must be displaced. This is achieved with a rapid 10 mL flush with normal saline. The initial flush will be met with inherent resistance as the fibrin mesh is being displaced.

Initial experience with using semi-automated intraosseus devices is very encouraging: they have been shown to be rapid and effective for obtaining circulatory access (Eisenkraft *et al.*, 2007; Brenner *et al.*, 2008; Horton & Beamer, 2008; Frascone *et al.*, 2009).

Resuscitation medications

In this section, medications used in paediatric resuscitation will be discussed. Calculating paediatric doses in the emergency situation is difficult, and it is advisable to have a paediatric chart (see Fig. 2.2) or similar to refer to.

Adrenaline

Adrenaline is administered routinely in most resuscitation attempts every 3–5 minutes. It improves coronary and cerebral blood flow (Schleien *et al.*, 1986). It also increases the vigour and intensity of VF, which may contribute to successful defibrillation (Otto *et al.*, 1981). Because acidosis and hypoxaemia can depress the action of adrenaline (Huang *et al.*, 1995), it is important to ensure that effective ventilations and chests compressions are continued.

The recommended dose is 10 μg/kg (0.1 mL/kg of 1:10 000 solution, with a maximum of 1 mg for a single dose), repeated every 3–5 minutes for ongoing arrest (Resuscitation Council (UK), 2011). If the child is in a shockable rhythm, adrenaline administration is delayed until after the third shock.

The tracheal tube route is no longer advocated, but if it is used, 100 μg/kg (0.1 mL/kg of 1:1000 solution) is recommended. However, the resulting plasma concentrations are unpredictable (Kleinman *et al.*, 1999).

Atropine

The most likely cause of bradycardia in infants and children is hypoxia. Initial treatment therefore involves ensuring adequate ventilation and oxygenation; if drug therapy is required, adrenaline is usually the first-line medication (Biarent et al., 2010).

Atropine is sometimes administered for symptomatic bradyarrhythmias, particularly if they have been induced by vagal stimulation during suction, tracheal intubation or cholinergic drug toxicity. If administered, the recommended dose of atropine is 20 μg/kg intravenously. As small doses of atropine can cause paradoxical bradycardia, a minimum dose of 100 μg is recommended.

Amiodarone

Amiodarone should be considered in refractory VF/pulseless VT after the third shock. The recommended dose is 5 mg/kg administered by a rapid intravenous bolus. It may be repeated after the fifth shock if required.

Calcium

The routine use of calcium does not improve the outcome from cardiac arrest (Stueven *et al.*, 1985a, 1985b). It may have detrimental effects in the ischaemic myocardium and may impair cerebral recovery. Specific indications for its use include:

- Hypocalcaemia – which is relatively common in critically ill children, particularly in septicaemia (Cardenas- Rivero *et al.*, 1989)
- Hyperkalaemia (Bisogno *et al.*, 1994)
- Hypermagnesaemia (Advanced Life Support Group, 2011)
- Calcium channel blocker overdose

The dose is 0.2 mL/kg of 10% calcium chloride intravenously. Careful administration is required as extravasation around the cannula may cause severe tissue injury. It should not be administered simultaneously with sodium bicarbonate via the same route.

Sodium bicarbonate

Although sodium bicarbonate has traditionally been administered for the treatment of severe metabolic acidosis associated with cardiac arrest, it has not been shown to improve outcome (Levy, 1998). In addition, there are numerous detrimental side-effects including:

- The generation of carbon dioxide
- An exacerbation of intracellular acidosis
- Impaired oxygen delivery to the tissues (Bellingham *et al.*, 1971)
- Metabolic alkalosis
- Hypernatraemia (Aufderheide *et al.*, 1992)
- Hyperosmolality (Bishop & Weisfeldt, 1976)

Respiratory failure is the major cause of cardiac arrest in children. As sodium bicarbonate raises carbon dioxide tension, its administration in a paediatric arrest may in fact worsen existing respiratory acidosis. Consequently, the initial priorities in paediatric resuscitation are attention to effective ventilation and quality chest compressions.

Indications for considering administering sodium bicarbonate include (Resuscitation Council (UK), 2011):

- Prolonged cardiac arrest
- Severe metabolic acidosis that has contributed to the arrest

If administered, the recommended dose for sodium bicarbonate is 1 mmol/kg (1 mL/kg of 8.4% solution, giving 2 mL/kg of 4.2% solution in infants under 3 months of age; Resuscitation Council (UK), 2011). A flush with 0.9% sodium chloride should always precede and follow administration (as sodium bicarbonate can inactivate other drugs). Care should be taken as extravasation may cause severe tissue injury.

Adequate ventilation must be maintained to avoid respiratory acidosis (the bicarbonate ion being excreted as carbon dioxide via the lungs). The blood pH and base excess should also be monitored, although the accuracy of arterial blood gas analysis during cardiac arrest or severe shock has been questioned.

Magnesium

Indications for administering magnesium include:

- Hypomagnesaemia (Biarent *et al.*, 2010)
- Torsades de pointes VT (Banai & Tzivoni, 1993)

The recommended dose is 25–50 mg/kg (to a maximum of 2 g) in a rapid intravenous infusion over several minutes (Advanced Life Support Group, 2011).

Fluids

If the cardiac arrest has resulted from circulatory failure, a standard bolus of 20 mL/kg 0.9% sodium chloride should be administered. This will probably need to be repeated.

Blood administration is recommended in children with severe haemorrhage who have not responded to 40 mL/kg of crystalloid (Resuscitation Council (UK), 2011).

Glucose

Infants and children have high glucose requirements (particularly when they are seriously ill) and low glycogen stores. However, it is not known whether the administration of glucose improves the cardiac function and survival of hypoglycaemic children in cardiac arrest. The routine use of glucose in resuscitation is therefore not recommended, except when documented hypoglycaemia is present (Biarent *et al.*, 2010). If glucose is required, the recommended dose is 200 mg/kg glucose (2 mL/kg 10% glucose; Resuscitation Council (UK), 2011).

Hyperglycaemia should also be avoided as it will increase cerebral metabolism and may have detrimental effects on neurological outcome. In addition, hyperglycaemia will cause a sharp rise in serum osmolality, which may result in osmotic diuresis.

Potential reversible causes of cardiac arrest

As it is rare for infants and children to have a primary cardiac arrest, it is important to identify and treat the initial cause of the cardiorespiratory collapse. The search for, and treatment of, potentially reversible causes of cardiac arrest is paramount, particularly when PEA is present. These causes can conveniently be classified into two groups for ease of memory – four 'Hs' and four 'Ts':

- Hypoxia
- Hypovolaemia
- Hyper/hypokalaemia/metabolic disturbance
- Hypothermia
- Tension pneumothorax
- Tamponade (cardiac)
- Toxins
- Thromboemboli

If an underlying cause is detected, it should be treated rapidly and appropriately. The treatment of these causes will now be briefly discussed.

Hypoxia

Hypoxia is a common cause of cardiorespiratory arrest in children. Effective ventilation with 100% oxygen is recommended in all paediatric cardiac arrests. This will help to correct hypoxia if it is present and will prevent it occurring. If the child is intubated, the mnemonic DOPES (see Chapter 5) is worth considering.

Hypovolaemia

Causes could include severe haemorrhage and severe diarrhoea and vomiting. Intravascular volume should be restored using appropriate fluids, and urgent surgical referral should be arranged if haemorrhage suspected. Circulatory volume replacement starting with 20 mL/kg of normal saline 0.9% stat.

Hyper/hypokalaemia/metabolic disturbance

The diagnosis of electrolyte and metabolic disorders can be confirmed by laboratory tests, although the child's history, e.g. renal disease, may be suggestive of abnormal blood chemistry. If possible, the disorder should be corrected. Calcium is usually administered if hyperkalaemia is suspected or confirmed (Bisogno *et al.*, 1994). Hypoglycaemia and hyperglycaemia are commonly associated with paediatric resuscitation; the child's blood glucose should be closely monitored and problems corrected (Biarent *et al.*, 2010).

Hypothermia

Hypothermia is rarely a problem in hospitalised children. However, it should be particularly suspected following an immersion injury. Small and premature infants are particularly susceptible to hypothermia. A low-reading thermometer should be used, and if necessary the child should be rapidly rewarmed (see Chapter 10).

Tension pneumothorax

Possible causes of a tension pneumothorax include chest trauma, asthma, thoracic surgery and central venous (subclavian) cannulation. Clinical features include decreased air entry, chest movement and hyperresonance on the affected side; the trachea may be deviated away from the affected side (Resuscitation Council (UK), 2011).

Needle thoracocentesis (into the mid-clavicular line in the second intercostal space on the affected side) with a wide-bore cannula is the standard initial treatment, followed by the insertion of a chest drain.

Tamponade (cardiac)

Cardiac tamponade occurs when blood or other fluids fill up the pericardial space, raising the intrapericardial pressure, compressing the heart and preventing it from filling. Causes include chest trauma and cardiothoracic surgery (Advanced Life Support Group, 2011).

Clinical features include distended neck veins, hypotension and muffled heart sounds. Unfortunately, these can be obscured by the cardiac arrest itself. Initially, needle pericardiocentesis is performed to relieve the tamponade.

Toxins

If there is no specific history related to toxins (accidental or deliberate, therapeutic or toxic), the cause may only be established following laboratory investigations (Resuscitation Council (UK), 2011). Where applicable, the appropriate antidote should be administered. Treatment is often only supportive.

Thromboembolism

Although very rare, if a pulmonary embolism is suspected, an emergency pulmonary embolectomy may be required. If possible, the child should be transferred to a cardiovascular surgical department. Thrombolysis will need to be considered.

Summary

In this chapter, the Resuscitation Council's PALS algorithm has been outlined. The principles of intraosseous infusion have been discussed, together with the use of resuscitation drugs. The treatment of potential reversible causes of paediatric cardiac arrest has been outlined.

References

Abdelmoneim, T., Kissoon, N., Johnson, L., *et al.* (1999) Acid-base status of blood from intraosseous and mixed venous sites during prolonged cardiopulmonary resuscitation and drug infusions. *Critical Care Medicine*, **27**, 1923–1928.

Advanced Life Support Group (2011) *Advanced Paediatric Life Support*, 5th edn. Wiley Blackwell, Oxford.

Andropoulos, D.B., Soifer S.J. & Schreiber, M.D. (1990) Plasma epinephrine concentrations after intraosseous and central venous injection during cardiopulmonary resuscitation in the lamb. *Journal of Pediatrics*, **116**, 312–315.

Aufderheide, T., Martin, D., Olson, D., *et al.* (1992) Prehospital bicarbonate use in cardiac arrest: a 3-year experience. *American Journal of Emergency Medicine*, **10**, 4–7.

Banai, S. & Tzivoni, D. (1993) Drug therapy for torsades de pointes. *Journal of Cardiovascular Electrophysiology*, **4**, 206–210.

Bellingham, A., Detter, J. & Lenfant, C. (1971) Regulatory mechanisms of hemoglobin oxygen affinity in acidosis and alkalosis. *Journal of Clinical Investigation*, **50**, 700–706.

Berg, R.A. (1984) Emergency infusion of catecholamines into bone marrow. *American Journal of Diseases in Children*, **138**, 810.

Biarent, D., Bingham, R., Christoph, E., *et al.* (2010) European Resuscitation Council Guidelines for Resuscitation Section 6. Paediatric life support (2010) *Resuscitation*, **81**, 1364–388.

Bishop, R. & Weisfeldt, M. (1976) Sodium bicarbonate administration during cardiac arrest: effect on arterial pH, PCO2 and osmolality. *JAMA*, **235**, 506–509.

Bisogno, J., Langley, A. & Von Dreele, M. (1994) Effect of calcium to reserve the electrocardiographic effects of hyperkalaemia in the isolated rat heart: a prospective, dose-response study. *Critical Care Medicine*, **22**, 697–704.

Brenner, T., Bernhard, M., Helm, M., *et al.* (2008) Comparison of two intraosseous infusion systems for adult emergency medical use. *Resuscitation*, **78**, 314–319.

Brickman, K., Krupp, K., Rega, P., *et al.* (1992) Typing and screening of blood from intraosseous access. *Annals of Emergency Medicine*, **21**, 414–417.

Cardenas-Rivero, N., Chernow, B., Stoiko, M., *et al.* (1989) Hypocalcaemia in critically ill children. *Journal of Pediatrics*, **114**, 946–951.

Eisenkraft, A., Gilat, E., Chapman, S., *et al.* (2007) Efficacy of the bone injection gun in the treatment of organophosphate poisoning. *Biopharmaceutical and Drug Disposition*, **28**, 145–150.

Frascone, R., Jensen, J., Wewerka, S. & Salzman, J. (2009) Use of the pediatric EZ-IO needle by emergency medical services providers. *Pediatric Emergency Care*, **25**, 329–332.

Fuchs, S., LaCovey, D. & Paris, P. (1991) A prehospital model of intraosseous infusion. *Annals of Emergency Medicine*, **20**, 371–374.

Glaeser, P.W. & Losek, J.D. (1986) Emergency intraosseous infusions in children. *American Journal of Emergency Medicine*, **4**, 34–36.

Glaeser, P.W., Losek, J.D. & Nelson, D.B. (1988) Pediatric intraosseous infusions: impact on vascular access time. *American Journal of Emergency Medicine*, **6**, 330–332.

Heinild, S., Sodergaard, T. & Tudvad, F. (1974) Bone marrow infusions in childhood: experiences of 1000 infusions. *Journal of Pediatrics*, **30**, 400–412.

Horton, M.A. & Beamer, C. (2008) Powered intraosseous insertion provides safe and effective vascular access for pediatric emergency patients. *Pediatric Emergency Care*, **24**, 347–350.

Huang, Y., Wong, K., Yip, W., *et al.* (1995) Cardiovascular responses to graded doses of three catecholamines during lactic and hydrochloric acidosis in dogs. *British Journal of Anaesthesia*, **74**, 583–590.

Johnson, L., Kissoon, N., Fiallos, M., *et al.* (1999) Use of intraosseous blood to assess blood chemistries and hemoglobin during cardiopulmonary resuscitation with drug infusions. *Critical Care Medicine*, **27**, 1147–1152.

Kleinman, M., Oh, W. & Stonestreet, B. (1999) Comparison of intravenous and endotracheal epinephrine during electromechanical dissociation with CPR in dogs. *Annals of Emergency Medicine*, **27**, 2748–2754.

La Fleche, F., Slepin, M., Vargas, J. & Milzman, D. (1989) Iatrogenic bilateral tibial fractures after intraosseous infusion attempts in a 3 month old infant. *Annals of Emergency Medicine*, **18**, 1099–1101.

Levy, M. (1998) An evidence-based evaluation of the use of sodium bicarbonate during cardiopulmonary resuscitation. *Critical Care Medicine*, **14**, 457–483.

McNamara, R.M., Spivey, W.H., Unger, H.D. & Malone, D.R. (1987) Emergency applications of intraosseous infusion. *Journal of Emergency Medicine*, **5**, 97–101.

Otto, C., Yakaitis, R. & Blitt, C. (1981) Mechanism of action of epinephrine in resuscitation from asphyxial arrest. *Critical Care Medicine*, **9**: 321–324.

Quan, L., Graves, J., Kinder, D., *et al.* (1992) Transcutaneous cardiac pacing in the treatment of out-of-hospital pediatric cardiac arrests. *Annals of Emergency Medicine*, **21**, 905–909.

Resuscitation Council (UK) (2011) *Paediatric Immediate Life Support*, 2nd edn. Resuscitation Council (UK), London.

Rosetti, V., Thompson, B., Miller, J., *et al.* (1985) Intraosseous infusion: an alternative route of pediatric intravascular access. *Annals of Emergency Medicine*, **14**, 885–888.

Rosovsky, M., FitzPatrick, M., Goldfarb, C. & Finestone, H. (1994) Bilateral osteomyelitis due to intraosseous infusion: case report and review of the English-language literature. *Pediatric Radiology*, **24**, 72–73.

Schleien, C.L., Dean, J.M. & Koehler, R.C. (1986) Effect of epinepherine on cerebral and myocardial perfusion in an infant animal preparation of cardiopulmonary resuscitation. *Circulation*, **73**, 809–817.

Simmons, C., Johnson, N., Perkin, R. & van Stralen, D. (1994) Intraosseous extravasation complication reports. *Annals of Emergency Medicine*, **23**, 363–366.

Stueven, H., Thompson, B., Aprahamian, C., *et al.* (1985a) Lack of effectiveness of calcium chloride in refractory asystole. *Annals of Emergency Medicine*, **14**, 630–632.

Stueven, H., Thompson, B., Aprahamian, C., *et al.* (1985b) Lack of effectiveness of calcium chloride in refractory electromechanical dissociation. *Annals of Emergency Medicine*, **14**, 626–629.

Ummenhofer, W., Frei, F.J., Urwyler, A. & Drewe, J. (1994) Are laboratory values in bone marrow aspirate predictable for venous blood in paediatric patients? *Resuscitation*, **27**, 123–128.

Vidal, R., Kissoon, N. & Gayle, M. (1993) Compartment syndrome following intraosseous infusion. *Pediatrics*, **91**, 1201–1202.

Voelckel, W.G., Lindner, K.H., Wenzel, V., *et al.* (2000) Intraosseous blood gases during hypothermia: correlation with arterial, mixed venous, and sagittal sinus blood. *Critical Care Medicine*, **28**, 2915–2920.

Chapter 9

Management of Anaphylaxis

Introduction

Anaphylaxis is an acute, severe hypersensitivity reaction that can lead to asphyxia, cardiovascular collapse and cardiac arrest. Its incidence is on the increase (Department of Health, 2006), probably associated with a notable increase in the prevalence of allergic diseases over the last 30 years (Working Group of the Resuscitation Council (UK), 2008). It is often poorly managed; in particular, adrenaline is greatly underused.

Patients with anaphylaxis have life-threatening airway and/or breathing and/or circulatory problems usually associated with skin and mucosal changes, and should be recognised and treated following the Airway, Breathing, Circulation, Disability, Exposure (ABCDE) approach (Working Group of the Resuscitation Council (UK), 2008).

In 2008, the Resuscitation Council (UK) published its revised guidelines on the emergency treatment of anaphylaxis (Working Group of the Resuscitation Council (UK), 2008). The treatment of a child with anaphylaxis is essentially the same as that for an adult (Muraro *et al.*, 2007).

The aim of this chapter is for readers to understand the emergency treatment of anaphylaxis in children.

Paediatric Advanced Life Support: A Practical Guide for Nurses, Second Edition. Phil Jevon.
© 2012 Phil Jevon. Published 2012 by Blackwell Publishing Ltd.

Learning objectives

At the end of this chapter, the reader will be able to:

• Provide a definition of anaphylaxis
• Discuss the incidence of anaphylaxis
• Discuss the pathophysiology of anaphylaxis
• List the causes of anaphylaxis
• Describe the clinical features and diagnosis of anaphylaxis
• Discuss the treatment of anaphylaxis

Definition

Anaphylaxis can be defined as 'a severe, life-threatening, gener-alised or systemic hypersensitivity reaction' (Johansson *et al.*, 2004). Basically, it is a life-threatening allergic reaction – the extreme end of the allergic spectrum (Anaphylaxis Campaign, 2011).

The term 'anaphylactoid reaction' has previously been used to describe a severe allergic reaction that is not IgE-mediated; causes include aspirin, exercise and blood products. It is clinically indis-tinguishable from an anaphylaxis reaction (Jevon, 2004) and the term is no longer used (Resuscitation Council (UK), 2011a).

Incidence and mortality statistics

Incidence

The incidence of anaphylaxis is on the increase (Gupta *et al.*, 2007), probably associated with the notable increase in the prevalence of allergic diseases over the last 30 years (Working Group of the Resuscitation Council (UK), 2008). A review of the literature on the incidence of anaphylaxis shows the following (Working Group of the Resuscitation Council (UK), 2008; Jevon, 2009):

• The incidence of anaphylaxis in the general population has increased.
• Statistics from the American College of Allergy, Asthma and Immunology Epidemiology of Anaphylaxis Working Group show that the overall frequency of anaphylaxis episodes is

between 30 and 950 cases per 100 000 persons per year (Lieberman *et al.*, 2006).

- UK primary care data in 2005 show a lifetime age-standardised prevalence of a recorded diagnosis of anaphylaxis of 75.5 per 100 000 (Sheikh *et al.*, 2008); i.e. 1 in 1333 of the English population have suffered anaphylaxis at least once in their life (Working Group of the Resuscitation Council (UK), 2008).
- Since 1990, admissions for anaphylaxis have increased by 700% (Gupta *et al.*, 2007).
- In England, between 1990–91 and 2000–01, 13 230 individuals were admitted to hospital with anaphylaxis (Gupta *et al.*, 2003).
- Between 1991 and 1994, the number of discharges from hospitals in England with a diagnosis of anaphylaxis doubled from 415 to 876 (Sheikh & Alves, 2000).
- In 2004, 3171 patients were admitted to hospital with anaphylaxis (Peng & Jick, 2004).
- Anaphylaxis is more common in females than in males: in 2004, 58% of attendees to emergency departments with anaphylaxis were female and 42% were male (Peng & Jick, 2004). Webb & Lieberman (2006)'s findings were comparable: 62% females and 38% males.
- The mean age of patients with anaphylaxis is 37 years (Webb & Lieberman, 2006).
- Approximately 1 in 3500 emergency department attendances are due to anaphylaxis (Stewart & Ewan, 1996)
- 50% of all anaphylactic reactions in the community are treated in hospital, with 20% requiring admission (Uguz *et al.*, 2005).
- Recurrent anaphylaxis is estimated to occur in 1 in 12 people per year (Gupta *et al.*, 2004).

Mortality rates

In the UK, approximately 20 anaphylaxis-associated deaths are reported each year, although this could be a substantial underestimate (Working Group of Resuscitation Council (UK), 2008). Death from anaphylaxis is becoming more common, particularly in children and young adults (Ewan, 2000).

Overall, the prognosis of anaphylaxis is good, with a case fatality rate of less than 1% reported in most population-based studies (Yocum *et al.*, 1999; Brown *et al.*, 2001; Bohlke *et al.*, 2004). There is an increased risk of mortality associated with anaphylaxis in patients with pre-existing asthma, particularly if the asthma is poorly controlled or in those asthmatics who fail to use, or delay treatment with, adrenaline (Pumphrey & Gowland, 2007).

Pathophysiology

Irrespective of the mechanism of anaphylaxis, mast cells and basophils release histamines and other vasoactive mediators that produce circulatory, respiratory, gastrointestinal and cutaneous effects (Wyatt *et al.*, 2006). These effects can include the development of pharyngeal and laryngeal oedema, bronchospasm, decreased vascular tone and capillary leak causing circulatory collapse (Jevon, 2004).

Causes

Causes of anaphylaxis include (Working Group of the Resuscitation Council (UK), 2008; Anaphylaxis Campaign, 2011):

- Drugs, e.g. penicillin, aspirin and anaesthetics
- Bee/wasp stings
- Foods, e.g. peanuts, tomatoes and fish
- Blood products
- Immunisations
- Latex
- Contrast media
- Drugs, e.g. antibiotics and aspirin

Food is a very common cause of anaphylaxis in children (Alves & Sheikh, 2001). In approximately 40% of anaphylactic reactions, the cause is unknown (idiopathic anaphylaxis) (Webb & Lieberman, 2006; Greenberger, 2007).

Clinical features and diagnosis

The lack of a consistent clinical picture can sometimes make an accurate diagnosis difficult (Project Team of the Resuscitation

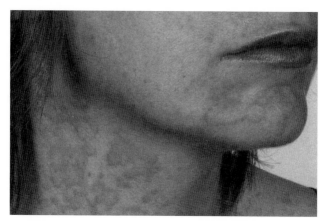

Fig. 9.1 Urticaria.

Council (UK), 2011a). Anaphylaxis can vary in severity, and the process can be slow, rapid or biphasic; occasionally, the onset may be delayed by a few hours and even persist for longer than 24 hours (Fisher, 1986). A detailed history and examination is essential as soon as possible. The clinical presentation often includes (Working Group of the Resuscitation Council (UK), 2008; Anaphylaxis Campaign, 2011):

- Urticaria (Fig. 9.1)
- Angioedema
- Respiratory distress
- Wheeze/stridor
- Cardiovascular shock
- Tachycardia and hypotension
- Pallor

The clinical features will vary depending on the cause, for example:

- *Ingested allergen (e.g. peanut)* – usually lip, mucosal and laryngeal oedema together with bronchoconstriction (Clarke & Nasser, 2001)
- *Injected or systemic allergens (e.g. insect venom or contrast media)* – usually hypotension
- *Allergen absorbed through the skin (e.g. latex)* – a slow onset as the allergen has to be absorbed through the skin (Ewan, 1998)

Anaphylaxis can vary in severity, and the onset is usually rapid, although it may occasionally be delayed by a few hours and even persist for longer than 24 hours (Fisher, 1986). The patient feels unwell, usually has skin changes, e.g. urticaria and angioedema, and will have a compromised airway and/or breathing and/or circulation (Jevon, 2008). Death from anaphylaxis usually occurs within 10–15 minutes, with cardiovascular collapse the most common cause of death (Resuscitation Council (UK), 2011a).

It is possible to mistake a panic attack or a vasovagal attack for anaphylaxis, and adrenaline has been administered inappropriately in these situations (Johnston *et al.*, 2003). The clinical features for both these presentations are as follows (Jevon, 2006):

- *A panic attack* – hyperventilation, tachycardia and anxiety-related erythematous rash, but no hypotension, pallor, wheeze or urticarial rash.
- *A vasovagal attack* – the absence of a rash, tachycardia and dyspnoea should rule out anaphylaxis as the cause of the collapse.

Measurement of mast cell tryptase levels is the specific test to confirm the diagnosis of anaphylaxis (Working Group of the Resuscitation Council (UK), 2008):

- *Minimum* – one sample 1–2 hours after the start of the symptoms
- *Ideal* – three time samples: as soon as is feasibly possible after the start of the symptoms, 1–2 hours after the start of the symptoms, and 24 hours later (or in the allergy clinic); serial samples are preferable

Treatment of anaphylaxis

The Resuscitation Council (UK) algorithm for the treatment of anaphylaxis in adults is detailed in Fig. 9.2. The treatment of anaphylaxis is as follows (Working Group of the Resuscitation Council (UK), 2008; Resuscitation Council (UK), 2011b):

1. Assess the child following the ABCDE approach described in Chapter 3.
2. Request expert help.

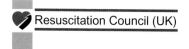
Resuscitation Council (UK)

Anaphylaxis algorithm

Anaphylactic reaction?

Airway, Breathing, Circulation, Disability, Exposure

Diagnosis - look for:
- Acute onset of illness
- Life-threatening Airway and/or Breathing and/or Circulation problems [1]
- And usually skin changes

- **Call for help**
- Lie patient flat
- Raise patient's legs

Adrenaline [2]

When skills and equipment available:
- Establish airway
- High flow oxygen
- IV fluid challenge [3]
- Chlorphenamine [4]
- Hydrocortisone [5]

Monitor:
- Pulse oximetry
- ECG
- Blood pressure

---

[1] **Life-threatening problems:**
Airway: swelling, hoarseness, stridor
Breathing: rapid breathing, wheeze, fatigue, cyanosis, SpO_2 < 92%, confusion
Circulation: pale, clammy, low blood pressure, faintness, drowsy/coma

---

[2] **Adrenaline** (give IM unless experienced with IV adrenaline)
IM doses of 1:1000 adrenaline (repeat after 5 min if no better)
- Adult   500 micrograms IM (0.5 mL)
- Child more than 12 years: 500 micrograms IM (0.5 mL)
- Child 6 -12 years: 300 micrograms IM (0.3 mL)
- Child less than 6 years: 150 micrograms IM (0.15 mL)

Adrenaline IV to be given **only by experienced specialists**
Titrate: Adults 50 micrograms; Children 1 microgram/kg

[3] **IV fluid challenge:**
Adult - 500 – 1000 mL
Child - crystalloid 20 mL/kg

Stop IV colloid
if this might be the cause
of anaphylaxis

---

	[4] Chlorphenamine (IM or slow IV)	[5] Hydrocortisone (IM or slow IV)
Adult or child more than 12 years	10 mg	200 mg
Child 6 - 12 years	5 mg	100 mg
Child 6 months to 6 years	2.5 mg	50 mg
Child less than 6 months	250 micrograms/kg	25 mg

See also: ▶ Anaphylactic reactions – Initial treatment

Fig. 9.2 Resuscitation Council (UK) anaphylaxis algorithm. Reproduced with the kind permission of the Resuscitation Council (UK).

3. If able, stop or remove the probable cause of the anaphylaxis; e.g. if a blood transfusion is in progress, stop it.
4. Recline the child into a position of comfort (the supine position may be helpful in hypotension but unhelpful in respiratory distress).
5. Ensure that the child has a clear airway. If stridor is present, alert senior expert help immediately (in anaphylaxis, stridor is probably due to potentially life-threatening laryngeal oedema).
6. Administer high-flow oxygen (15 L per minute) using a non-rebreather mask. Establish oxygen saturation monitoring using a pulse oximeter.
7. Insert a cannula. Commence intravenous fluids as a 20 mL/kg bolus of 0.9% normal saline, and repeat if necessary.
8. Establish continuous ECG monitoring – cardiac arrhythmias can sometimes occur (Resuscitation Council (UK), 2011a).
9. Closely monitor the child's vital signs.
10. Assess and reassess the patient following the ABCDE approach.
11. Repeat the adrenaline after 5 minutes if there is no improvement, Several doses may be required.
12. Do not sit or stand the child up if he is feeling faint or dizzy – he may be in profound shock and may then have a cardiac arrest.

Adrenaline

Adrenaline is the most important drug in anaphylaxis (Fisher, 1995). To be effective, it needs to be administered promptly (Patel *et al.*, 1994). Adrenaline:

- Reverses peripheral vasodilatation
- Reduces oedema
- Dilates the airways
- Increases myocardial contractility
- Suppresses histamine and leukotriene release

The recommended dose of adrenaline in children is as follows:

- <6 years of age –150 µg intramuscularly (0.15 mL 1:1000)
- 6–12 years – 300 µg intramuscularly (0.3 mL 1:1000)
- >12 years – 500 µg intramuscularly (0.5 mL 1:1000)

Adrenaline can be repeated after 5 minutes if there is no clinical improvement (Resuscitation Council (UK), 2011b); several doses may be required (see the *British National Formulary*). The intramuscular route for the administration of adrenaline is generally used as it is relatively safe and adverse effects are rare. The only severe adverse effect following intramuscular administration of adrenaline that has been reported has been a myocardial infarction in a patient with severe ischaemic heart disease (Saff *et al.*, 1993).

If the child has been prescribed an EpiPen Jnr or EpiPen or similar (Working Group of the Resuscitation Council (UK), 2008):

- EpiPen Jnr (150 µg) can be administered in children from 6 months to 6 years of age (instead of 120 µg)
- EpiPen (300 µg) can be administered instead in children over 6 years old (instead of 250 µg or 500 µg)

Additional fixed-dose self-administration syringes would facilitate more accurate dosing in young children (Simmons *et al.*, 2002).

The more hazardous intravenous route is occasionally used, particularly if the child is in profound shock that is judged to be immediately life-threatening or in certain situations such as anaesthesia (Working Group of the Resuscitation Council (UK), 2008). However, adrenaline administered intravenously can cause life-threatening cardiac arrhythmias, hypertension and myocardial ischaemia and is for specialist use only, e.g. anaesthetists, emergency physicians and intensive care doctors (Working Group of the Resuscitation Council (UK), 2008).

If an experienced specialist has chosen to administer the adrenaline intravenously, it is recommended that the dose of adrenaline is titrated according to the weight of the child (1 µg/kg, which is 0.01 mL/kg of 1:10 000 solution; Resuscitation Council (UK), 2011b). An adrenaline infusion may need to be started (Working Group of the Resuscitation Council (UK), 2008). The patient should be on a cardiac monitor, and resuscitation equipment should be immediately available.

Cautions include the following:

- Two strengths of adrenaline are available: 1:1000 solution is used for intramuscular injection, while 1:10 000 solution is used for intravenous injection (Jevon, 2008).
- The subcutaneous route for the administration of adrenaline should not be utilised because absorption is considerably slower (Jevon, 2009).

Intravenous fluid challenge

If severe hypotension is present, a fluid challenge is recommended: 500–1000 mL of a crystalloid solution, e.g. 0.9% normal saline, is suitable. Further infusion may be required (Working Group of the Resuscitation Council (UK), 2008).

Chlorpheniramine

Chlorpheniramine (Piriton) should be used routinely for all anaphylactic reactions. Its use may be beneficial and is unlikely to be harmful (Working Group of the Resuscitation Council (UK), 2008). Care should be taken to avoid drug-induced hypotension. The recommended doses are as follows:

- <6 months of age: 250 µg /kg intramuscularly or slowly intravenously
- 6 months – 6 years: 2.5 mg intramuscularly or slowly intravenously
- 6–12 years: 5 mg intramuscularly or slowly intravenously
- >12 years: 10 mg intramuscularly or slowly intravenously

Hydrocortisone

Hydrocortisone should be administered following severe anaphylaxis to help prevent late sequelae, particularly in asthmatics who have previously been on corticosteroidal treatment (Resuscitation Council (UK), 2011a). The recommended dose is 200 mg either intramuscularly or by slow intravenous injection, and care should be taken to avoid inducing further hypotension (Working Group of the Resuscitation Council (UK), 2008).

- <6 months of age: 25 mg intramuscularly or slowly intravenously
- 1–6 years: 50 mg intramuscularly or slowly intravenously
- 6–12 years: 100 mg intramuscularly or slowly intravenously
- >12 years: 200 mg intramuscularly or slowly intravenously

Inhaled beta-2-agonist

Consider further bronchodilatory therapy, e.g. salbutamol (inhaled or intravenously; Working Group of the Resuscitation Council (UK), 2008).

Cardiac arrest following anaphylaxis

All the principles of basic and advanced life support apply to a patient with an anaphylaxis-induced cardiac arrest (Resuscitation Council (UK), 2005). In particular:

- Secure the airway with a tracheal tube as soon as possible – senior anaesthetic help will undoubtedly be required, particularly if laryngeal and/or pharyngeal oedema is present
- Administer adrenaline intravenously and not intramuscularly
- Provide aggressive fluid resuscitation if shock was present prior to collapse

Follow-up

Even if the reaction is only moderate, the patient should be warned of the possibility of an early recurrence of symptoms. Monitoring for 8–24 hours is sometimes required, particularly when the reaction (Jevon, 2004):

- Is severe and is of slow onset due to idiopathic anaphylaxis
- Occurs in a patient who is severely asthmatic
- Is complicated by a severe asthmatic attack
- Could again be triggered again because further absorption of the allergen is possible

Referring the child to an allergy clinic is essential. The cause of the anaphylaxis can be established by taking a structured allergy history and confirmed by the presence of specific IgE antibodies identified by skin prick tests or a specific challenge to confirm or exclude the diagnosis (Clarke & Nasser, 2001).

Advice should be given concerning allergen avoidance. This is backed up by educating the parents or carers and relevant school personnel (Ewan & Clark, 2001). Where appropriate, this should include the effective administration of adrenaline via an autoinjector device. The wearing of a MedicAlert bracelet may be required.

Summary

Anaphylaxis can be life-threatening. This chapter has detailed the guidelines issued by the Resuscitation Council (UK) to treat it (Working Group of the Resuscitation Council (UK), 2008). Early treatment with intramuscular adrenaline is paramount.

References

Alves, B. & Sheikh, A. (2001) Age specific aetiology of anaphylaxis. *Archives of Disease in Childhood*, **85**, 348.

Anaphylaxis Campaign: www.anaphylaxis.org.uk (accessed 3 June 2011).

Bohlke, K., Davis, R.L., DeStefano, F., *et al.* (2004) Epidemiology of anaphylaxis among children and adolescents enrolled in a health maintenance organization. *Journal of Allergy and Clinical Immunology*, **113**, 536–542.

Brown, A.F., McKinnon, D. & Chu, K. (2001) Emergency department anaphylaxis: a review of 142 patients in a single year. *Journal of Allergy and Clinical Immunology*, **108**, 861–866.

Clarke, A. & Nasser, S. (2001) *Anaphylaxis. Continuing Medical Focus: The state of Allergy/Immunotherapy in UK*. Rita Publications, London.

Department of Health (2006) *A Review of Services for Allergy. The Epidemiology, Demand for, and Provision of Treatment and Effectiveness of Clinical Interventions*. Department of Health, London.

Ewan, P. (1998) ABC of allergies: Anaphylaxis. *BMJ*, **316**, 1442.

Ewan, P. (2000) Anaphylaxis. In *ABC of Allergies* (ed. S. Durham). BMJ Books, London.

Ewan, P. & Clark, A. (2001) Long-term prospective observational study of patients with peanut and nut allergy after participation in a management plan. *Lancet*, **357**, 111.

Fisher, M. (1986) Clinical observations on the pathophysiology and treatment of anaphylactic cardiovascular collapse. *Anaesthesia and Intensive Care*, **14**, 17–21.

Fisher, M. (1995) Treatment of acute anaphylaxis. *BMJ*, **311**, 731–733.

Greenberger, P. (2007) Idiopathic anaphylaxis. *Immunology and Allergy Clinics of North America*, **27**, 273–293.

Gupta, R., Sheikh, A., Strachan, D. & Anderson, H. (2003) Increasing hospital admissions for systemic allergic disorders in England: an analysis of national admissions data. *BMJ*, **327**, 1142–1143.

Gupta, R., Sheikh, A., Strachan, D.P. & Anderson, H. (2004) Burden of allergic disease in the UK: secondary analyses of national databases. *Clinical and Experimental Allergy*, **34**, 520–526.

Gupta, R., Sheikh, A., Strachan, D. & Anderson, H. (2007) Time trends in allergic disorders in the UK. *Thorax*, **62**, 91–96.

Jevon, P. (2004) *Anaphylaxis: A Practical Guide*. Butterworth Heinemann, Oxford.

Jevon, P. (2006) An overview of managing anaphylaxis in the community. *Nursing Times*, **102**, 48.

Jevon, P. (2008) Severe allergic reaction: management of anaphylaxis in hospital. *British Journal of Nursing*, **17**, 104–108.

Jevon, P. (2009) *Advanced Cardiac Life Support*, 2nd edn. Wiley Blackwell, Oxford.

Johansson, S., Bieber, T., Dhal, R., *et al.* (2004) Revised nomenclature for allergy for global use: report of the Nomenclature Review Committee of the World. *Journal of Allergy and Clinical Immunology*, **11**, 832-836.

Johnston, S., Unsworth, J. & Gompels, M. (2003) Adrenaline given outside the context of life-threatening allergic reactions. *BMJ*, **326**, 589–590.

Lieberman, P., Camargo, C., Jr., Bohlke, K. *et al.* (2006) Epidemiology of anaphylaxis: findings of the American College of Allergy, Asthma and Immunology Epidemiology of Anaphylaxis Working Group. *Annals of Allergy, Asthma and Immunology*, **97**, 596–602.

Muraro, A., Roberts, G., Clark, A., *et al.* (2007) The management of anaphylaxis in childhood: position paper of the European Academy of Allergology and Clinical Immunology. *Allergy*, **62**, 857–871.

Patel, L., Radivan, F.S. & David, T.J. (1994) Management of anaphylactic reactions to food. *Archives of Disease in Childhood*, **71**, 370–375.

Peng, M. & Jick, H. (2004) A population based study of the incidence, cause and severity of anaphylaxis in the United Kingdom. *Archives of Internal Medicine*, **164**, 317–319.

Project Team of the Resuscitation Council (UK) (2005) *Emergency Medical Treatment of Anaphylactic Reactions*. Resuscitation Council (UK), London.

Pumphrey, R. & Gowland, M. (2007) Further fatal allergic reactions to food in the United Kingdom, 1999–2006. *Journal of Allergy and Clinical Immunology*, **119**, 1018–1019.

Resuscitation Council (UK) (2011a) *Advanced Life Support*, 6th edn. Resuscitation Council (UK), London.

Resuscitation Council (UK) (2011b) *Paediatric Immediate Life Support*, 2nd edn. Resuscitation Council (UK), London.

Saff, R., Nahhas, A. & Fink, J. (1993) Myocardial infarction induced by coronary vasospasm after self-administration of epinephrine. *Annals of Allergy*, **70**, 396–398.

Sheikh, A. & Alves, B. (2000) Hospital admissions for acute anaphylaxis: time trend study. *BMJ*, **320**, 1441.

Sheikh, A., Hippisley-Cox, J., Newton, J. & Fenty, J. (2008) Trends in national incidence, lifetime prevalence and adrenaline prescribing for anaphylaxis in England. *Journal of the Royal Society of Medicine*, **101**, 139–143.

Simmons, F., Gu, X., Silver, N. & Simmons, K. (2002) EpiPen Jr versus EpiPen in young children weighing 15–30kg at risk of anaphylaxis. *Journal of Allergy and Clinical Immunology*, **109**, 171–175.

Stewart, A. & Ewan, P. (1996) The incidence, aetiology and management of anaphylaxis presenting to an Accident & Emergency Department. *Quarterly Journal of Medicine*, **89**, 859–864.

Uguz, A., Lack, G., Pumphrey, R., *et al.* (2005) Allergic reactions in the community: a questionnaire survey of members of the anaphylaxis campaign. *Clinical and Experimental Allergy*, **35**, 746–750.

Webb, L. & Lieberman, P. (2006) Anaphylaxis: a review of 601 cases. *Annals of Allergy, Asthma and Immunology*, **97**, 39–43.

Working Group of the Resuscitation Council (UK) (2008) *Emergency Treatment of Anaphylactic Reactions: Guidelines for Healthcare Providers*. Resuscitation Council (UK), London.

Wyatt, J., Illingworth, R., Graham, C., *et al.* (2006) *Oxford Handbook of Emergency Medicine*, 3rd edn. Oxford University Press, Oxford.

Yocum, M., Butterfield, J., Klein, J., *et al.* (1999) Epidemiology of anaphylaxis in Olmsted County: a population-based study. *Journal of Allergy and Clinical Immunology*, **104**(2 Pt 1), 452–456.

Further resources

Allergy UK: www.allergyuk.org

Chapter 10

Resuscitation in Special Situations

Introduction

Resuscitation in certain special situations, e.g. hypothermia, requires modification to the standard basic life support (BLS) and advanced life support (ALS) guidelines in order to optimise the chances of survival. These situations are often suspected from the history surrounding the event, a knowledge of the common causes of cardiac arrest in the various age groups or prompt results from diagnostic investigations.

The aim of this chapter is to provide an understanding of the principles of resuscitation in special situations.

Learning objectives

At the end of the chapter, the reader will be able to discuss the principles of cardiac management associated with the following special situations:

- Epiglottitis
- Hypothermia
- drowning
- Acute severe asthma
- Electrocution
- Poisoning
- Trauma

Paediatric Advanced Life Support: A Practical Guide for Nurses, Second Edition.
Phil Jevon.
© 2012 Phil Jevon. Published 2012 by Blackwell Publishing Ltd.

Epiglottitis

Epiglottitis is a potentially life-threatening condition. Character-ised by severe swelling of the epiglottitis and surrounding tissues, it is usually caused by infection with *Haemophilus influenzae* type B (Resuscitation Council (UK), 2006). It is now quite rare because of the HiB vaccination in infancy (although it may still occur in cases where the vaccine has failed and in unimmunised children (Advanced Life Support Group, 2011). It is mainly seen in chil-dren aged 1–6 years, but it can occur both in infants and in adults (Advanced Life Support Group, 2011).

Pre-arrest

Typical clinical features of epiglottitis include:

- An acute onset
- Lethargy
- Pyrexia
- Pallor
- Sitting still with the chin raised, the mouth open and excessive drooling (as the child is unable to swallow saliva)
- A gradual increase in respiratory distress, possibly with associ-ated stridor
- Reluctance to talk

Treatment

Movement, change of position, attempts to look in the child's mouth, attempts to cannulate, etc. can all make the child worse and can even lead to complete obstruction of the airway. It is important to leave the child with the parents.

Expert help will be required as soon as possible because the child will need to be intubated under controlled conditions (Resuscitation Council (UK), 2006). Because of intense swelling and inflammation of the epiglottis ('cherry red epiglottis'), tra-cheal intubation may be difficult; it will be necessary to use a smaller tracheal tube than would normally be used for the child's size (Advanced Life Support Group, 2011).

Once the airway has been secured, blood should be sent for culture, and intravenous antibiotics (cefotaxime or ceftriaxone) should be commenced (Advanced Life Support Group, 2011). The prognosis is then excellent.

Cardiac arrest

If a child with epiglottitis has a cardiac arrest, begin ventilation with a bag-valve-mask device (ensure that the pressure relief valve has been overriden), and await expert help. The child will need urgent tracheal intubation – a surgical airway may be needed (Resuscitation Council (UK), 2006).

Hypothermia

> Hypothermia can mimic death, and death can mimic hypothermia.

Classification

Hypothermia can be defined as a core body temperature of less than 35 °C. It can be classified (Resuscitation Council (UK), 2011) as:

- Mild (>32 – <35 °C)
- Moderate (30–32 °C)
- Severe (<30 °C)

Physiological effects of hypothermia

Severe hypothermia is associated with a marked fall in cerebral blood flow and oxygen requirements, reduced cardiac output and decreased arterial pressure (Schneider, 1992). If there is rapid cooling prior to the development of hypoxaemia, decreased oxygen consumption and metabolism may precede the cardiac arrest and reduce organ ischaemia (Larach, 1995), exerting a protective effect on the brain and vital organs during cardiac arrest (Holzer *et al.*, 1997).

Core temperature-related cardiac arrhythmias – sinus bradycardia, atrial fibrillation, ventricular fibrillation (VF) and finally asystole – can complicate hypothermia (Resuscitation Council (UK), 2011).

If the core temperature is less than 30 °C, defibrillation is unlikely to be effective until rewarming has been accomplished (Advanced Life Support Group, 2011). In the presence of hypothermia, the heart may not respond to cardioactive drugs and pacemaker stimulation. The metabolism of drugs is reduced, and following repeated administration, drug levels can rise to toxic values (Resuscitation Council (UK), 2011).

Rewarming

Rewarming at a rate of 0.25–0.5 °C per hour is recommended (Advanced Life Support Group, 2011) until a core temperature of 32–34 °C has been achieved (Resuscitation Council (UK), 2006).

External rewarming methods

External rewarming methods are usually adequate if the core temperature is over 30 °C (Advanced Life Support Group, 2011). Practical options include warm blankets, a warm air system and a heating blanket. Remove wet, cold clothing if necessary.

Core rewarming methods

Core rewarming methods should be used in a child with a core temperature of less than 30 °C (Advanced Life Support Group, 2011). Methods include (Advanced Life Support Group, 2011):

- Intravenous fluids warmed up to 39 °C
- Ventilator gases warmed up to 42 °C
- Gastric or bladder lavage with normal saline at 42 °C
- Peritoneal lavage with potassium-free dialysate at 42 °C, giving 20 mL/kg with a 15 minute cycle
- Pleural or pericardial lavage
- Endovascular warming
- Extracorporeal blood rewarming (the preferred option in a cardiac arrest)

Although passive rewarming methods, e.g. warm blankets or a warm environment, may suffice in cases of mild hypothermia, they will be ineffective if the patient is in cardiac arrest (Larach, 1995).

Physiological effects of rewarming

The process of rewarming can cause vasodilatation and an expansion of the vascular space. Large volumes of fluid may need to be administered. In addition, severe hyperkalaemia may also develop, which will need correcting.

Resuscitation

All the principles of BLS and ALS apply to the hypothermic child (Biarent *et al.*, 2010). However, some modifications to the approach are required:

- Ventilate with warmed (40–46 °C) and humidified oxygen – intubate the patient as soon as possible.
- Confirm hypothermia using a low-reading thermometer once cardiopulmonary resuscitation (CPR) has been started.
- Prevent further heat loss if possible, e.g. remove wet clothing.
- Begin core rewarming method(s) as facilities and expertise allow (see below).
- In shock-refractory VF/VT (i.e. when the first three shocks are unsuccessful), defer further defibrillation attempts until the core temperature has reached over 30 °C (Resuscitation Council (UK), 2011).
- Provide fluid resuscitation as required.
- Withhold drugs until the core temperature is over 30 °C. Then double the standard time intervals between drug administration and use the lowest recommended drug doses. Follow standard drug protocols *only* once the core temperature is returning towards normal (Resuscitation Council (UK), 2011).
- Handle the child carefully – rough movement can precipitate cardiac arrhythmias.
- Do not confirm death until the child's core temperature is at least 32 °C or until efforts to raise the core temperature have failed (Advanced Life Support Group, 2011). Prolonged CPR will usually be required.

Drowning

Death from drowning is the third most common cause of accidental death in the paediatric age group in the UK (after road traffic accidents and burns), and often occurs in private swimming pools, garden ponds and other inland waterways (Advanced Life Support Group, 2011).

Although survival is rare following a prolonged submersion and a prolonged resuscitation attempt, successful resuscitation associated with full neurological recovery is still possible in these circumstances. If submersion occurs in icy water, the rapid development of hypothermia can provide some cerebral protection from hypoxia, particularly in small children (Quan & Kinder, 1992).

The most significant and detrimental consequence of submersion is hypoxia, the duration of which is a critical factor in determining the patient's outcome (Resuscitation Council (UK), 2006). Oxygenation, ventilation and perfusion are therefore of paramount importance.

Clearing the airways of aspirated water is not necessary (Rosen *et al.*, 1995). Approximately 10–15% of patients develop intense laryngeal spasm, which protects the lungs from aspiration of water or gastric contents (Skinner & Vincent, 1997). Even if water is aspirated, this is only likely to be in small amounts, and it is rapidly absorbed into the central circulation (Rosen *et al.*, 1995). Vomiting or regurgitation of the gastric contents is common (Manolios & Mackie, 1988).

Prognostic indicators

Responsiveness, either at the scene or on arrival at the A&E department, is a good prognostic indicator (Cummings & Quan, 1999). Poor prognostic indicators following submersion in children and adolescents include (Quan & Kinder, 1992):

- A duration of submersion of over 25 minutes
- A duration of resuscitation of over 25 minutes
- Pulseless cardiac arrest on arrival at the A&E department
- Severe acidosis
- The presence of VF/VT on the first recorded ECG.

Resuscitation

All the principles of BLS and ALS apply when undertaking CPR on a child following submersion. However, some modifications to the approach are required:

- If cervical spine injury is suspected (e.g. the incident was associated with diving or water slide use), apply a jaw thrust, rather than a head tilt–chin lift, to open the airway, and immobilise the child's spine using a cervical collar and spinal board or equivalent (Resuscitation Council (UK), 2006).
- Insert a nasogastric tube. Empty and decompress the stomach – there is a risk of aspiration (Advanced Life Support Group, 2011).
- Administer antibiotics if there are signs of infection (which are more likely following submersion in a river)

In addition the child may be hypothermic. The problems associated with undertaking CPR in the presence of hypothermia, together with specific modifications to the standard BLS and ALS protocols including rewarming, have already been discussed (see above). Wet clothing should be removed.

Acute severe asthma

Acute severe asthma attacks are normally reversible, and related deaths should be considered avoidable (Resuscitation Council (UK), 2011). They are 10 times more common at night (Brenner *et al.*, 1998), and most asthma-related deaths occur outside hospital. National guidelines recommend aggressive treatment of acute severe asthma (oxygen, a beta-2-agonist, e.g. salbutamol, corticosteroids and aminophylline) to prevent deterioration to cardiac arrest.

Causes of cardiac arrest associated with acute severe asthma include:

- Severe bronchospasm and mucous plugging
- Hypoxia-related cardiac arrhythmias
- Tension pneumothorax

Resuscitation

All the principles of BLS and ALS apply to undertaking CPR in a patient suffering a cardiac arrest following an acute severe asthma attack. However, some modifications to the approach are required:

- Intubate the trachea as soon as possible because high resistance in the airways can hinder ventilation. High ventilation pressures are usually required, and gastric distension usually occurs during bag-valve-mask ventilation.
- Ensure prolonged inspiratory and expiratory times (8–10 inflations per minute) if necessary, in order to avoid high intrinsic positive end-expiratory pressure. A complication of this is sudden severe hypotension (Resuscitation Council (UK), 2011).
- Dynamic hyperventilation will increase transthoracic impedance (Deakin *et al.*, 1998), so when it is present consider higher defibrillation energies if initial defibrillation attempts are unsuccessful (Resuscitation Council (UK), 2011).

Note that the high airway pressures required for ventilation can cause a tension pneumothorax. Clinical features include unilateral chest wall expansion, tracheal displacement to the opposite side and subcutaneous emphysema (Resuscitation Council (UK), 2011).

Electrocution

Electrocution can result from domestic or industrial electricity, or from a lightening strike. Children account for about a third of all victims of electrocution (Advanced Life Support Group, 2011). Electrocution injuries in children mainly occur at home and are associated with a low-voltage current (Resuscitation Council (UK), 2011).

Lightening strike injuries have a mortality rate of 30%, with 70% of those who survive sustaining significant morbidity (Stewart, 2000). Worldwide lightening strikes cause 1000 deaths each year (MMWR, 1998). Injury can also occur indirectly through ground current from current splashing from a tree or similar object that has been struck by lightening (Zafren *et al.*, 2005).

Factors affecting severity of the injury

Factors affecting the severity of electrical injury include the magnitude of the energy delivered, voltage, resistance to current flow, type of current, duration of contact with the source of the current and current pathway (Resuscitation Council (UK), 2006).

Skin resistance, the most important factor impeding the flow of current, is reduced significantly by moisture, turning a minor injury into a life-threatening one (Wallace et al, 1995).

Types of current

There are two types of current:

- *Direct current (DC)* – this is present in batteries and in lightening. The current flows in one direction for the duration of the discharge. This induces one strong muscular contraction that often throws the casualty away from the current source (Fontanarosa, 1993). Asystole is more common after a DC shock (Resuscitation Council (UK), 2011)
- *Alternating current (AC)* – this is present in most household and commercial sources of electricity. Contact with it may cause tetanic skeletal muscle contractions, preventing self-release from the current source (Resuscitation Council (UK), 2011). The repetitive frequency of AC increases the risk of current flow through the myocardium during the vulnerable refractory period of the cardiac cycle, which can cause VF (Geddes *et al.*, 1986).

Transthoracic current flow (a hand-to-hand current pathway) is more likely to be fatal than is a vertical current pathway (hand to foot) or a straddle current pathway (foot to foot) (Thompson & Ashwal, 1983).

Clinical effects on the child

Electrocution injuries result from the direct effects of the current on cell membranes and vascular smooth muscle, and the production of heat energy as the current passes through the body tissues (Resuscitation Council (UK), 2011).

Cardiac arrest, VF or asystole is the primary cause of death following electrocution. Respiratory arrest can be caused by a variety of different mechanisms (Resuscitation Council (UK), 2011):

- Passage of electric current through the brain inhibiting the respiratory centre in the medulla

- Tetanic contraction of the diaphragm and chest wall during exposure to the current
- Prolonged paralysis of the respiratory muscles

Electrical injuries often cause related trauma, e.g. cervical spine injury (Epperley & Stewart, 1989), and skin burns.

Resuscitation

All the principles of BLS and ALS apply to undertaking CPR in a patient suffering a cardiac arrest following electrocution (Resuscitation Council (UK), 2006). However, some modifications to the approach are required:

- If applicable, ensure that the environment is safe and there is no electrocution risk to the team.
- Immobilise the cervical spine and apply a jaw thrust (rather than head tilt–chin lift) to open the airway.
- Intubate early, particularly if there are burns to the face, mouth or neck (as soft tissue oedema may rapidly develop and obstruct the airway) (Resuscitation Council (UK), 2006).
- As muscular paralysis may persist for several hours following electrocution (Kleinschmidt-Demasters, 1995), monitor the breathing and provide assisted ventilation as required (Resuscitation Council (UK), 2006).
- Remove any smouldering clothes or shoes to prevent further thermal injury.
- Administer sufficient fluids to maintain adequate diuresis to excrete the byproducts of tissue production, including potassium and myoglobin (Cooper, 1995).
- Continue CPR for prolonged periods if required.
- Request surgical expertise if there are severe thermal injuries.

Poisoning

Poisoning is a leading cause of cardiac arrest in the under-40-year-old age group (Watson *et al.*, 2004; Resuscitation Council (UK), 2006). Long-term survival following a cardiac arrest associated with poisoning is approximately 24% (Resuscitation Council (UK), 2011).

Death from poisoning in the paediatric age group is on the decline, particularly following the introduction of child-resistant drug containers in the 1970s (although 20% of children under 5 years can open them!; Advanced Life Support Group, 2011). However, suspected poisoning still accounts for approximately 40 000 attendances at A&E departments in England and Wales each year (Advanced Life Support Group, 2011).

With some poisoning agents, cardiac arrest results from direct cardiotoxicity, while with others it is secondary to respiratory arrest caused by central nervous system depression or aspiration of gastric contents. Pulseless electrical activity, a common complication of ingesting drugs with negative inotropic properties, carries a far better prognosis than when associated with a primary cardiac cause (Resuscitation Council (UK), 2011).

The emphasis is on intensive supportive therapy and correcting hypoxia, acid–base and electrolyte disorders (Resuscitation Council (UK), 2006).

Prevention of cardiac arrest

Prevention of cardiorespiratory arrest is a priority: follow the ABCDE approach to assess and treat the patient (Resuscitation Council (UK), 2011) while waiting for the poison to be eliminated (Zimmerman, 2003). Particular attention to maintaining a clear airway and adequate breathing is required; a decreased level of consciousness can be associated with poisoning that can lead to a compromised airway and inadequate ventilation, resulting in cardiorespiratory arrest and death (not uncommon) (Resuscitation Council (UK), 2011).

Specific therapeutic measures

As stated above, the emphasis is ongoing intensive supportive therapy, correcting hypoxia, acid–base and electrolyte disorders. Very few therapeutic therapies are helpful (Resuscitation Council (UK), 2011). However, the following may be considered.

Activated charcoal
Although it can absorb certain drugs, the value of activated charcoal decreases over time, and there is no evidence that it improves survival (Resuscitation Council (UK), 2011).

A single dose of activated charcoal is recommended when a potentially toxic amount of poison (one which is known to be absorbed by activated charcoal) has been ingested less than 60 minutes previously (Chyka *et al.*, 2005). Repeated doses may be helpful in life-threatening poisoning with carbamazepine, phenobarbital, quinine, theophylline or dapsone (Resuscitation Council (UK), 2011).

Activated charcoal must not be administered unless the child can maintain his own airway or the airway is secured with a tracheal tube.

Gastric lavage

This is only useful if the poison has been ingested less than 60 minutes previously, and generally only following tracheal intubation (Resuscitation Council (UK), 2011). Delayed gastric lavage is not helpful and may in fact push the poison further down the gastrointestinal tract (Vale & Kulig, 2004).

Whole-bowel irrigation

This can be useful in some situations, e.g. a potentially toxic ingestion of certain sustained-release or enteric medications and iron, or the removal of packets containing illicit drugs (Resuscitation Council (UK), 2006).

Haemodialysis

Haemodialysis can be useful for eliminating life-threatening drugs or metabolites that are water soluble, have a low volume of distribution and low plasma protein binding, e.g. methanol or salicylates (Golper & Bennett, 1988).

Specific antidotes

Administer specific antidotes as necessary (consultation with TOXBASE may be required). Commonly used antidotes are discussed below.

Antidote for opiates (including methadone)

The clinical features of opiates poisoning include respiratory depression, pinpoint pupils and unconsciousness. Naloxone remains the treatment of choice to reverse narcotic toxicity. The recommended dose is 0.1 mg/kg intravenously (to a maximum of 2 mg in one dose). Care should be taken to ensure adequate ventilation prior to the administration of naloxone because ventricular arrhythmias may occur in the presence of hypercapnia (Osterwalder, 1996). As the action of naloxone lasts for approximately 45–70 minutes, compared with several hours for opiates (Resuscitation Council (UK), 2011), repeated doses may be required.

Antidotes for tricyclic antidepressants
Poisoning with tricyclic antidepressants can lead to convulsions and cardiac arrhythmias. Toxicity can result in preterminal sinus bradycardia and atrioventricular block with junctional or ventricular broad-complex escape beats. A QRS complex greater than 0.16 seconds (four small squares) is considered to be a predictor of serious toxicity (Advanced Life Support Group, 2011). Most life-threatening complications occur within 6 hours of ingestion.

Alkalisation (to a pH of at least 7.45 and ideally 7.50) is recommended because it will reduce the toxic effects on the heart; this can be achieved by hyperventilation and the administration of sodium bicarbonate (1–2 mmol/kg intravenously; Advanced Life Support Group, 2011). Sodium bicarbonate can also help to suppress cardiac arrhythmias and reverse hypotension.

If the cardiac arrhythmias do not respond to the sodium bicarbonate, an antiarrhythmic drug may be required. However, guidance from a poisons unit is advisable because some antiarrhythmics are contraindicated in this situation.

Convulsions should be treated, initially with lorazepam 0.1 mg/kg intravenously (or rectal diazepam if intravenous access cannot be secured; Advanced Life Support Group, 2011). Hypotension should be treated initially with fluid resuscitation 20 mL/kg.

Cardiopulmonary resuscitation
All the principles of BLS and ALS apply to undertaking CPR in a patient suffering a cardiac arrest following poisoning (Resuscitation Council (UK), 2006). Some modifications to the approach are, however, required:

- If necessary, ensure that relevant precautions are taken if poisoning is due to gas, corrosives, etc.
- Intubate the patient as soon as possible as poisoning is associated with a high incidence of pulmonary aspiration of gastric contents.

- If possible, identify the poison(s) ingested: information from the patient's relatives and friends and ambulance crew may be of help. Also examine the patient for needle puncture marks, tablet bottles/sachets, odours and corrosion around the mouth.
- Access TOXBASE or telephone the National Poisons Information Service if specialist help and advice is required.
- Continue CPR for prolonged periods if required as the poison may be metabolised or excreted during this time (Resuscitation Council (UK), 2006)

Trauma

Poor resuscitation technique is a major cause of preventable death associated with paediatric trauma (McKoy & Bell, 1983). Common contributing factors include failure to:

- Open and maintain a clear airway
- Provide appropriate fluid resuscitation with a head injury
- Recognise and treat internal haemorrhage

Causes of cardiac arrest in a child with trauma include hypoxia, tension pneumothorax, hypovolaemia and cardiac tamponade.

Resuscitation

All the principles of BLS and ALS apply to undertaking CPR in a patient suffering a cardiac arrest following trauma. Some modifications to the approach are, however, required:

- Perform a jaw thrust and not a head tilt–chin lift to open the airway.
- Immobilise the cervical spine – which is difficult in young children when trying to maintain the head in the neutral position. Cervical spine injury is less common in children than in adults. It is more commonly associated with road traffic accidents and falls from a height.
- Exclude tension pneumothorax when ventilating.
- Site two wide-bore cannulae and administer volume replacement if indicated – a transfusion of 10–15 mL/kg of blood may be required.

- Request surgical expertise and treat any life-threatening problems.
- Suspect thoracic injury (as there is often no external evidence) if there is a history of thoracoabdominal trauma or if ventilation is difficult.

Life-threatening electrolyte abnormalities

Life-threatening electrolyte abnormalities, e.g. hypokalaemia and hyperkalaemia, can cause cardiac arrhythmias and cardiac arrest.

Hypokalaemia

Hypokalaemia can be defined as a serum potassium of less than 3.5mmol/L (Wyatt *et al.*, 2006). Severe hypokalaemia (<2.5mmol/L) may cause life-threatening cardiac arrhythmias. Causes include (Resuscitation Council (UK), 2011):

- Diarrhoea leading to gastrointestinal loss
- Endocrine disorders, e.g. Cushing syndrome
- Metabolic acidosis
- Hypomagnesaemia
- Dialysis

Treatment of hypokalaemia (<2.5mmol/L or cardiac arrhythmias present)
Administer potassium 0.5mmol/kg per hour via an intravenous infusion until the serum potassium reaches over 3.5mmol/L or the cardiac arrhythmias cease (Resuscitation Council (UK), 2006). The child should ideally be closely monitored on a paediatric intensive care unit or high-dependency unit.

Hypomagnesaemia is often associated with hypokalaemia (magnesium being important for the uptake of potassium and for the maintenance of intracellular potassium levels) (Resuscitation Council (UK), 2011). It is therefore recommended that magnesium stores should be replenished if hypokalaemia is severe (Cohn *et al.*, 2000).

Hyperkalaemia

Hyperkalaemia can be defined as a serum potassium of over 7 mmol/L (Resuscitation Council (UK), 2006). Causes include (Resuscitation Council (UK), 2006, 2011; Wyatt *et al.*, 2006):

- Renal failure leading to a fall in potassium excretion
- Adrenal insufficiency
- Acidosis
- Cell injury, e.g. rhabdomyolysis
- Following a massive blood transfusion

Depending on the severity of hyperkalaemia, the aims of treatment (Resuscitation Council (UK), 2011) are to:

- Protect the myocardium
- Move potassium into the cells
- Remove potassium from the body
- Monitor serum potassium levels in case rebound hyperkalaemia occurs
- Prevent recurrence

Treatment for hyperkalaemia in a child not in cardiac arrest
Treatment for hyperkalaemia depends on the speed of occurrence of the symptoms, together with the clinical state of the child or the presence of toxic changes on the ECG (Resuscitation Council (UK), 2006; Advanced Life Support Group, 2011):

- *Hyperkalaemia only (no symptoms, no ECG changes)* – diuretics, salbutamol (see Box 10.1 for the dose to be administered via a nebuliser), potassium exchange resin (calcium resonium 1 g/kg orally or rectally), sodium bicarbonate (1–2 mmol/kg intravenously) and haemodialysis (or peritoneal dialysis)

Box 10.1 Doses of nebulised salbutamol for hyperkalaemia (Advanced Life Support Group, 2011)

- <2.5 years: 2.5 mg
- 2.5–7 years: 5 mg
- >7 years: 10 mg

- *Hyperkalaemia and symptoms or toxic ECG changes* – calcium chloride intravenously over 2–5 minutes, sodium bicarbonate (if acidosis or renal failure is present; 1–2 mmol/kg intravenously), an insulin–glucose infusion (glucose 10% 5 mL/kg and insulin 0.05 U/kg per hour intravenously) and haemodialysis

Treatment for hyperkalaemia in a child in cardiac arrest

There are no modifications to BLS and ALS. The initial specific treatment usually involves administering calcium chloride intravenously or intraorally to antagonise the toxic effects of hyperkalaemia at the myocardial cell membrane.

Hypercalcaemia and hypocalcaemia

Hypocalcaemia

Hypocalcaemia can complicate any serious illness, particularly septicaemia (Advanced Life Support Group, 2011). The signs and symptoms may include weakness, tetany, convulsions, hypotension and cardiac arrhythmias (Resuscitation Council (UK), 2006). Although treatment is aimed at the underlying clinical condition, intravenous calcium may be indicated (a bolus followed by an infusion) in an emergency situation (Advanced Life Support Group, 2011).

Hypercalcaemia

Hypercalcaemia, which usually presents as long-standing anorexia, malaise, weight loss, failure to thrive and vomiting, has a number of causes, including hyperparathyroidism, hypervitaminosis D or A, idiopathic hypercalcaemia of infancy, malignancy, thiazide diuretic abuse and skeletal disorders (Advanced Life Support Group, 2011). Fluid resuscitation is the initial treatment in the emergency situation (Resuscitation Council (UK), 2006).

Summary

Resuscitation in certain special situations requires modification to the standard BLS and ALS guidelines if the chances of survival are to be optimised. The key principles of resuscitation in these special situations have been discussed.

References

Advanced Life Support Group (2011) *Advanced Paediatric Life Support*, 5th edn. Wiley Blackwell, Oxford.

Biarent, D., Bingham, R., Christoph, E., *et al.* (2010) European Resuscitation Council Guidelines for Resuscitation Section 6. Paediatric life support (2010) *Resuscitation*, **81**, 1364–1388.

Brenner, B. & Kohn, M. (1998) The acute asthmatic patient in the ED: to admit or discharge. *American Journal of Emergency Medicine*, **16**, 69–75.

Chyka, P., Seger, D., Krenzelok, E. & Vale, J. (2005) Position paper: single-dose activated charcoal. *Clinical Toxicology*, **43**, 61–87.

Cohn, J., Kowey, P., Whelton, P. & Prisant, L. (2000) New guidelines for potassium replacement in clinical practice: a contemporary review by the National Council on potassium in Clinical Practice. *Archives of Internal Medicine*, **160**, 2429–2436.

Cooper, M. (1995) Emergency care of lightening and electrical injuries. *Seminars in Neurology*, **15**, 268–278.

Cummings, P. & Quan, L. (1999) Trends in unintentional drowning: the role of alcohol and medical care. *JAMA*, **281**, 2198–2202.

Deakin, C., McLarren, R., Petley, G. *et al.* (1998) Effects of positive end-expiratory pressure on transthoracic impedance – implications for defibrillation. *Resuscitation*, **37**, 9–12.

Epperley, T. & Stewart, J. (1989) The physical effects of lightening injury. *Journal of Family Practice*, **29**, 267–272.

Fontanarosa, P. (1993) Electrical shock and lightning strike *Ann Emerg Med*, **22**, 378–387.

Geddes, L., Bourland, J. & Ford, G. (1986) The mechanism underlying sudden death from electric shock. *Medical Instrumentation*, **20**, 303–315.

Golper, T.A. & Bennett, W.M. (1988) Drug removal by continuous arteriovenous haemofiltration – a review of the evidence in poisoned patients. *Medical Toxicology and Adverse Drug Experience*, **3**, 341–349.

Holzer, M., Behringer, W., Schorkhuber, W., *et al* (1997) Mild hypothermia and outcome after CPR. Hypothermia for Cardiac Arrest (HACA) Study Group. *Acta Anaesthesiologia Scandinavica Supplementum*, **111**, 55–58.

Kleinschmidt-DeMasters, B. (1995) Neuropathology of lightening strike injuries. *Seminars in Neurology*, **15**, 323–328.

Larach, M. (1995) Accidental hypothermia. *Lancet*, **345**, 493–498.

McKoy, C. & Bell, M. (1983) Preventable traumatic deaths in children. *Journal of Pediatric Surgery*, **18**, 505–508.

Manolios, N. & Mackie, I. (1988) Drowning and near-drowning on Australian beaches patrolled by life-savers: a 10-year study, 1973–1983. *Medical Journal of Australia*, **148**: 165–167, 170–171.

MMWR (1998) Lightening associated deaths – United States 1980–1995. *MMWR Morbidity and Mortality Weekly Reports*, **47**, 391–394.

Osterwalder, J. (1996) Naloxone: for intoxications with intravenous heroin and heroin mixtures: harmless or hazardous? *Journal of Toxicology. Clinical Toxicology*, **34**, 409–416.

Quan, L. & Kinder, D. (1992) Pediatric submersions: prehospital predictors of outcome. *Pediatrics*, **90**, 909–913.

Resuscitation Council (UK) (2006) *European Paediatric Life Support*, 2nd edn. Resuscitation Council (UK), London.

Resuscitation Council (UK) (2011) *Advanced Life Support*, 6th edn. Resuscitation Council (UK), London.

Rosen, P., Stoto, M. & Harley, J. (1995) The use of the Heimlich maneuver in near-drowning: Institute of Medicine report. *Journal of Emergency Medicine*, **13**, 397–405.

Schneider, S. (1992) Hypothermia: from recognition to rewarming. *Emergency Medicine Reports*, **13**: 1–20.

Skinner, D. & Vincent, R. (1997) *Cardiopulmonary Resuscitation*, 2nd edn. Oxford University Press, Oxford.

Stewart, C. (2000) When lightening strikes. *Emergency Medical Services*, **29**: 57–67.

Thompson, J.C. & Ashwal, S. (1983) Electrical injuries in children. *Am J Dis Child*, **137**, 231–235.

Vale, J. & Kulig, K. (2004) Position paper: gastric lavage. *Clinical Toxicology*, **42**, 933–943.

Wallace, B., Cone, J., Vanderpool, R., *et al.* (1995) Retrospective evaluation of admission criteria for paediatric electrical injuries. *Burns*, **21**, 590–593.

Watson, W., Litovitz, T., Klein-Schwartz, W., *et al.* (2004) 2003 annual report of the American Association of Poison Control Centers Toxic exposure Surveillance system. *American Journal of Emergency Medicine*, **22**, 335–404.

Wyatt, J., Illingworth, R., Graham, C., Clancy, M. & Robertson, C. (2006) *Oxford Handbook of Emergency Medicine*, 3rd edn. Oxford University Press, Oxford.

Zafren, K., Durrer, B., Herry, J. & Brugger, H. (2005) Lightening injuries: prevention and on-site treatment in mountains and remote areas. Official guidelines of the International Commission for Mountain Emergency Medicine and the Medical Commission of the International Mountaineering and Climbing Federation (ICAR and UIAA MEDCOM). *Resuscitation*, **65**, 369–372.

Zimmerman, J. (2003) Poisonings and overdoses in the intensive care unit: general and specific management issues. *Critical Care Medicine*, **31**, 2794.

Chapter 11

Post-resuscitation Care

Introduction

After prolonged, complete, whole-body hypoxia-ischaemia, return of spontaneous circulation (ROSC) has been described as an unnatural pathophysiological state created by successful cardiopulmonary resuscitation (Nolan *et al.*, 2008). It is important that post-resuscitation care, which should be meticulously undertaken by a multidisciplinary team, includes all the treatments needed for complete neurological recovery (Briarent *et al.*, 2010). Following the ABCDE approach will help the team to focus on priorities (Resuscitation Council (UK), 2011).

The main goals of post-resuscitation care are to reverse brain injury and myocardial dysfunction, as well as to treat the systemic ischaemia/reperfusion response and any persistent precipitating pathology (Biarent *et al.*, 2010).

The aim of this chapter is to understand the principles of post-resuscitation care.

Learning objectives

At the end of this chapter, the reader will be able to:

- List the goals of post-resuscitation care
- Outline the initial assessment priorities following the ABCDE approach
- Describe measures to limit secondary cerebral damage

Paediatric Advanced Life Support: A Practical Guide for Nurses, Second Edition.
Phil Jevon.
© 2012 Phil Jevon. Published 2012 by Blackwell Publishing Ltd.

- Outline the guidelines for referral to a paediatric intensive care unit (PICU)
- Discuss the standards for the retrieval of critically ill children
- List the basic principles of safe transport

Goals of post-resuscitation care

The goals of post-resuscitation care are to:

- Perform an initial assessment of the child following the ABCDE approach
- Preserve cerebral function
- Limit damage to the vital organs
- Identify and treat the cause of illness
- Transfer the patient to definitive care in the best physiological state

Initial assessment and treatment priorities following the ABCDE approach

The initial management priorities involve opening and maintaining a clear airway, ensuring adequate ventilation and ensuring adequate circulation. The familiar ABCDE approach will help post-resuscitation care to focus on the priorities.

Airway

The child's airway may be at risk due to a reduced level of consciousness or a depressed gag reflex. Prompt assessment of the child's airway should therefore be undertaken: check the mouth (the signs and treatment of a partially or completely obstructed airway were discussed in detail in Chapter 3) and apply suction using a rigid wide-bore cannula (Yankauer) if required.

Check the child's level of consciousness. A tracheal tube may need to be inserted to secure the airway and facilitate mechanical ventilation. Correct tracheal tube placement, together with tube patency, should be verified and regularly monitored. If the clinical state of an intubated child deteriorates, remember the mnemonic DOPES, (see Chapter 5).

Breathing

Having ensured that the child's airway is secure, check the breathing. Inadequate ventilation leading to prolonged hypoxia will increase the risk of a further cardiac arrest and could contribute to further neurological damage. The child's breathing and ventilation status should therefore be accurately assessed and supported if necessary. Respiratory assessment was described in detail in Chapter 3.

Respiratory monitoring should initially include:

- *Pulse oximetry* – oxygen delivery titrated to achieve an oxygen saturation of between 94% and 98% (Resuscitation Council (UK), 2011)
- *Arterial blood gas analysis* – and acid–base measurement
- *Capnography* – which helps to avoid hypoventilation and hyperventilation (Tobias *et al.*, 1996)
- *Chest X-ray* – to check for any lung pathology or rib fractures, and to assess tracheal tube placement

If the child is not breathing adequately, mechanical ventilation should continue using the available equipment, e.g. a bag-valve device and portable ventilator. If a mechanical ventilator is being used, the recommended initial tidal volumes are 7–10 mL/kg, sufficient to achieve a visible chest rise and audible breath sounds over the distal lung fields (American Academy of Pediatrics, 2000).

Once there is ROSC, oxygen delivery should be titrated and guided by pulse oximetry in order to avoid the harmful effects of hyperoxaemia (Biarent *et al.*, 2010). The aim is to achieve oxygen saturation levels of 94–98% (Resuscitation Council (UK), 2011), except in anaemia and carbon monoxide poisoning, in which a high inspired oxygen concentration is recommended.

A nasogastric tube may need to be inserted to decompress the stomach (the gastric inflation often associated with bag-valve-mask ventilation can cause diaphragmatic splinting and allow aspiration of gastric contents).

Circulation

Circulatory dysfunction frequently occurs following resuscitation from cardiac arrest (Lucking *et al.*, 1986). Common causes include:

- Myocardial depression due to hypoxia, acidosis and toxins
- Hypovolaemia
- Acid–base disturbance
- Electrolyte abnormality
- Loss of peripheral vascular tone

The maintenance of an adequate cardiac output and oxygen delivery to the tissues is paramount if multiorgan function is to be preserved (American Academy of Pediatrics, 2000). Clinical assessment of circulation and cardiac output should therefore be carried out (see Chapter 3 for a detailed description of circulatory assessment).

Clinical signs of inadequate cardiac output and poor tissue perfusion include:

- Tachycardia
- A delayed capillary refill time (>2 seconds)
- Cool and pale peripheries
- Weak or absent distal pulses
- Decreased urine output
- Altered neurological status (e.g. confusion, agitation and a decrease in conscious level)
- Hypotension (a late sign)

Blood pressure may be normal despite the presence of shock.

The pulse should be noted and ECG monitoring started. Blood pressure measurements should be recorded, together with adequacy of peripheral perfusion (temperature, colour and capillary refill of the peripheries). The neurological status and urine output should also be closely monitored.

The insertion of an arterial cannula will allow continuous arterial blood pressure measurements and repeated sampling for arterial blood gas analysis. Central venous pressure monitoring may be required, and urine output should be closely monitored. A pulmonary artery may sometimes be inserted to monitor pulmonary capillary wedge pressure and cardiac output (Ceneviva *et al.*, 1998), although non-invasive Doppler techniques may be a better alternative.

Myocardial dysfunction is common following cardiopulmonary resuscitation (Hildebrand *et al.*, 1988; Checchia *et al.*, 2003; Mayr *et al.* 2007; Nolan *et al.*, 2008). Vasoactive drugs, e.g. adrenaline, dobutamine, dopamine and noradrenaline, can improve the child's post-arrest haemodynamic status, but it is important that they are titrated according to the clinical condition (Kern *et al.*, 1996; Meyer *et al.*, 2002; Vasquez *et al.*, 2004; Huang *et al.*, 2005a, 2005b; Studer *et al.*, 2005).

Disability

The child's blood glucose should be measured and monitored (see below).

A baseline neurological assessment should be undertaken and documented using the AVPU (Alert, Voice, Pain, Unresponsive) scale or the Glasgow Coma Score (GCS) or Paediatric GCS (for children under 4 years of age).

The GCS, originally developed to grade severity and outcome in traumatic head injury (Teasdale & Jennett, 1974), is now used as an unvalidated tool for the description of states of consciousness from all pathologies (Advanced Life Support Group, 2011). The GCS will provide a benchmark for further assessments. However, in the post-resuscitation phase, pupil size can be affected by carbon dioxide retention, adrenaline and local ischaemia at the front of the eye.

It is possible to minimise the risk of brain injury by stabilising the blood pressure, preventing/treating seizures, correctly any electrolyte abnormalities and normalising blood gases (Resuscitation Council (UK), 2011).

Exposure

It is important to undertake a complete examination of the child to detect any lesions, e.g. rashes, as this may help to confirm the diagnosis and may guide appropriate treatment and management (Resuscitation Council (UK), 2011).

Glucose control

Both hypoglycaemia and hyperglycaemia may impair the outcome for critically ill children and should therefore be avoided (Resuscitation Council (UK), 2011). Aggressive glucose monitoring and treatment may, however, be harmful (Treggiari *et al.*, 2008).

Although there is insufficient evidence to support or refute a specific management strategy for glucose control in children with ROSC following a cardiac arrest, it is appropriate to monitor blood glucose and avoid hypoglycaemia as well as sustained hyperglycaemia (Biarent *et al.*, 2010).

Temperature control

Hypothermia

Hypothermia is a common finding in a child following successful cardiopulmonary resuscitation (Hickey *et al.*, 2003), and central hypothermia (32–34 °C) may in fact be beneficial (Biarent *et al.*, 2010). Therapeutic hypothermia (32–34 °C) should be considered in ventilated patients (Resuscitation Council (UK), 2011).

Hyperthermia

Hyperthermia, common in the post-resuscitation period (Biarent *et al.*, 2010), is associated with a poor neurological outcome (Takino and Okada, 1991; Zeiner *et al.*, 2001; Takasu *et al.*, 2001), with the risk increasing for each degree of body temperature greater than 37 °C (Zeiner *et al.*, 2001). Antipyretics and/or active cooling measures are recommended (Resuscitation Council (UK), 2011).

Maintaining renal function

Renal perfusion should be maximised and renal tubular patency maintained by ensuring an adequate urine flow by:

- Maintaining adequate oxygenation
- Maintaining adequate cardiac output
- Administering (judiciously) diuretics if necessary to maintain a urine output of greater than 1 mL/kg per hour
- Correcting any electrolyte and acid–base imbalances

Measures to minimise secondary cerebral damage

One of the aims of post-resuscitation care is to prevent further (secondary) cerebral damage. This can be achieved by maintaining cerebral blood flow, achieving normal cellular homeostasis and reducing cerebral metabolic needs (Advanced Life Support Group, 2011). The Advanced Life Support Group (2011) has identified the following practical measures to minimise secondary cerebral damage:

- Maintain adequate oxygenation.
- Maintain an adequate circulation, using inotropes and fluids as necessary.
- Correct any electrolyte imbalances.
- Correct any acid–base disturbance.
- Normalise the blood sugar.
- Normalise the body temperature.
- Administer adequate analgesia and sedation.
- Control any convulsions.
- Reduce intracranial pressure.

Guidelines for referral to a paediatric intensive care unit

The Paediatric Intensive Care Society, in its Standards Document 2001, has issued guidelines for referral to a PICU. All purchasers and providers of healthcare and allied services should be aware of the guidelines for PICU referral. In addition, duty managers and consultants in all hospitals should be aware of how to contact the lead centre for paediatric intensive care. The guidelines are as follows:

- Intensive care admission must involve consultant-to-consultant referral between the consultant responsible for the patient's care in the referring centre and the consultant in charge of the PICU.
- The duty consultant in charge of PICU at the lead centre must be available for consultation at all times.

- Consultation between the referring unit and the lead centre must remain possible irrespective of whether an intensive care bed is available at the lead centre.
- The management of patients discussed with the lead centre remains the responsibility of the referring team until care has been taken over by a retrieval team or, in other circumstances, until after the patient has been transferred.
- Institutions without intensive care facilities on site should, by default, make all their paediatric intensive care referrals to a lead centre.
- Institutions with a paediatric or general intensive care unit that are not lead centres for paediatric intensive care should refer patients to the lead centre if intensive care is likely to be required for more than 24 hours, or if it is indicated because of failure or a need for support involving more than one organ system.
- Any decision to refer a patient outside the normal referral region for paediatric intensive care should involve consultation between the referring consultant and the consultant in charge of the lead centre.

Standards for retrieval of critically ill children

The Paediatric Intensive Care Society, in its Standards Document 2001, has made recommendations in respect of standards for the retrieval of critically ill children, as outlined below.

Applicability

- Lead centres should be funded for a retrieval service (24 hours a day, 7 days a week) for children who require intensive care within the agreed catchment area whenever they have an available bed.
- Supraregional transfer services should be separately funded as part of the funding of a supraregional service as distinct from a regional lead centre activity.
- In the presence of a separate, centralised designated paediatric intensive care retrieval service, the lead centre should ensure and endorse the standard and training of the staff providing the service.

- Centres providing supraregional services should have protocols in place for the transfer of such children from their referral centres.
- Primary transport (by referring hospitals) will be necessary for some conditions such as expanding intracranial haematoma and severe thoracic vascular trauma.
- Standards for primary transport (by referring hospitals) should be agreed with the lead centre or specialist unit, and the circumstances in which they should be used should be clearly defined.

Availability

- In normal circumstances, lead centres are obligated to retrieve patients referred and accepted for intensive care on their units. They are not obligated to transfer them elsewhere in the event of supraregional referral or a lack of available beds.
- The local lead centre retrieval service should be available on at least 95% of days, with a back-up plan for those occasions when the service is not available.
- In the presence of a separate, centralised designated paediatric intensive care retrieval service, this team should undertake the transfer of patients outside the normally served geographical region if required to do so for reasons of supraregional referral or lack of available beds.
- There should be equity of access to the retrieval service.

Medical staffing

- The retrieval service is staffed as a remote intensive care bed requiring one-to-one nursing and its own medical staff member.
- The service should be consultant-led and, where necessary, consultant-provided.
- During a retrieval performed by a paediatric intensive care consultant, the PICU should be covered by another paediatric intensive care consultant.
- The paediatric intensive care consultants from the lead centre are responsible for deciding which medical staff are appropriately trained and experienced to carry out retrieval and to agree the rota as appropriate.

- Training in paediatric intensive care transport must include supervised transports (i.e. accompanied by the trainer).
- The decision of what level of medical staff to despatch for retrieval should be made in consultation with the referring consultant and assessed as part of the referral for intensive care.
- In normal circumstances, if a primary transport is required (i.e. by staff from the referral hospital), the medical staff member involved must be appropriately trained, with general intensive care and paediatric airway expertise.

Nurse staffing

- The establishment for nursing at the lead centre should allow for a transport-trained nurse to be available to undertake retrieval duties 24 hours a day. They will therefore not be included in this baseline establishment.
- The lead nurse at the lead centre is responsible for deciding which nurses are appropriately trained and experienced to carry out retrieval and to agree the rota as appropriate. These are expected to be ENB 415 (or equivalent) trained.
- Training in paediatric intensive care transport must include supervised transports (i.e. accompanied by the trainer).
- If a primary transport is required (i.e. by staff from the referring hospital), the accompanying staff member involved must be a senior/experienced intensive care or A&E nurse or operating department practitioner.

Environment and support services

- Parents/carers should be given as much information about the retrieval service as early as possible at the referring centre.
- Parents/carers/guardians should be told that it is unlikely they will be able to accompany the child during transfer.
- Referring hospitals are obligated to provide transport to the lead centre for the parents of critically ill children being transferred.
- Advice about travel arrangements to the lead centre should be available for other family members.
- Wherever possible, the child should undergo only one retrieval journey.

Equipment and facilities

- The retrieval team should be able to retrieve the child from a designated critical care area within the referring hospital, which should be agreed with the lead centre.
- The retrieval team should be fully equipped and able to deal with children of all ages.
- Retrieval teams should not need to rely upon paramedic ambulance services.

Quality and management of services

- Compatible protocols should be developed between the lead centre and the referring hospitals.
- Arrangements for contacting the retrieval team should be clearly displayed within critical care areas at the referring hospitals.
- The lead centre must provide adequate information to the referring hospitals.
- The referring hospitals must undertake to provide full clinical information to the intended receiving team.
- The retrieval service should be continuously audited, and data collected on all referrals and retrievals. This includes referrals that do not result in transfer, and records should include the nature of any medical or nursing advice given by the lead centre.
- Critical incident recording should be included in retrieval records and audit.

Operational issues

Primary transport for emergencies such as neurosurgical intervention for an expanding intracranial haematoma should not be deferred or re-routed as a result of the actual, declared or suspected availability of a paediatric intensive care bed. The patient should be immediately transferred to the nearest centre capable of performing the life-saving procedure, and a paediatric intensive care bed should then be sought when the patient's condition has been stabilised, e.g. postoperatively.

By its very nature, retrieval exposes the staff (and patient) to additional personal and professional hazards. The service must be appropriately insured and indemnified, with written confirmation of such, before retrieval is offered. Furthermore, the establishment of a paediatric intensive care retrieval service has considerable implications for ambulance and other emergency services, which must be consulted during the planning and preparation phases of establishing a service. The likely modes of transport should be determined in advance, and their sources and availability identified and negotiated. Depending upon local circumstances and the nature of the individual case, the choice of vehicle may be different for the outward and return journeys.

In normal circumstances, paediatric intensive care retrieval is a 'secondary transfer' occurring with less desperate urgency than in a primary transfer after the patient has been resuscitated and stabilised. The retrieval service cannot provide timely assistance with the initial resuscitation. The onus of responsibility remains with the referring hospital to initiate and continue competent resuscitation and stabilisation from the outset until they hand over to the retrieval team.

The referral of a patient to a PICU must be on the basis of a referring consultant talking directly to the duty paediatric intensive care consultant.

There should be a dedicated telephone line on the PICU for arranging retrievals, the telephone number of which should be distributed to hospitals in the catchment area. Details of the patient's age, history, (likely) diagnosis, vital signs and precise location should be documented, along with a record of any advice given and contact telephone numbers.

Transport/retrieval staff must be skilled paediatric intensive care practitioners who have received specific additional training in transport as well as intensive care. The transport team should not be dependent upon paramedic support from the ambulance service.

A clear hierarchy among the retrieval team is necessary, with a single team leader designated. This individual is in charge of the patient, not the transport vehicle. Upon their arrival at the referring centre and after a concise but comprehensive medical and nursing handover, the team will take over clinical management and assume responsibility for the patient, who is then prepared for transport. The patient must not be moved until the retrieval team leader is satisfied that preparation for transport has been adequate.

Basic principles of safe transport

Meticulous attention to the initial assessment and resuscitation of the child, together with appropriate emergency management, will reduce the risk of transport-related morbidity and mortality (Advanced Life Support Group, 2011). Basic principles of safe transport apply to the movement of all sick children, whether within or between hospitals and whether or not a specialist retrieval team is involved, including:

- Stabilising the child prior to transport following the ABCDE approach (Henning, 1992; Resuscitation Council (UK), 2011)
- Securing the airway, ensuring adequate ventilation and adequate circulation
- Correcting any hypoglycaemia
- Securing intravenous lines, etc.
- Communicating effectively with the receiving hospital or department
- Communicating effectively with other members of the team
- Ensuring that adequate transport is arranged
- Organising appropriately trained staff to escort the patient
- Ensuring that appropriate emergency and monitoring equipment is assembled – all in working order, batteries fully charged, full oxygen cylinders, etc.
- Monitoring airway, breathing and circulation, and maintaining temperature (to prevent hypothermia)
- Ensuring that appropriate documentation is taken
- Ensuring adequate communication with the parents

Summary

Post-resuscitation care initially involves maintaining a clear airway, ensuring adequate ventilation and oxygenation with 100% oxygen, and ensuring adequate circulation. In addition, measures should be taken to minimise secondary cerebral damage. Guidelines for referral to a PICU and the standards for the retrieval of critically ill children have been discussed.

References

Advanced Life Support Group (2011) *Advanced Paediatric Life Support*, 5th edn. Wiley Blackwell, Oxford.

American Academy of Pediatrics (2000) *Pediatric Education for Prehospital Professionals*. Jones & Bartlett, Sudbury USA.

Biarent, D., Bingham, R., Christoph, E., *et al.* (2010) European Resuscitation Council Guidelines for Resuscitation Section 6. Paediatric life support (2010) *Resuscitation*, **81**, 1364–1388.

Ceneviva, G., Paschall, J., Maffei, F. & Carcillo, J. (1998) Hemodynamic support in fluid-refractory pediatric septic shock. *Pediatrics*, **102**: e19.

Checchia, P., Sehra, R., Moynihan, J., *et al.* (2003) Myocardial injury in children following resuscitation after cardiac arrest. *Resuscitation*, **57**, 131–137.

Henning, R. (1992) Emergency transport of critically ill children: stabilisation before departure. *Medical Journal of Australia*, **156**, 117–124.

Hickey, R., Kochanek, P., Ferimer, H., *et al.* (2003) Induced hyperthermia exacerbates neurologic neuronal histologic damage after asphyxial cardiac arrest in rats. *Critical Care Medicine*, **31**, 531–535.

Hildebrand, C.A., Hartmann, A.G., Arcinue, E.L., *et al.* (1988) Cardiac performance in pediatric near-drowning. *Critical Care Medicine*, **16**, 331–335.

Huang, L., Weil, M.H., Sun, S., *et al.* (2005a) Levosimendan improves postresuscitation outcomes in a rat model of CPR. *Journal of Laboratory and Clinical Medicine*, **146**, 256–261.

Huang, L., Weil, M., Tang, W., *et al.* (2005b) Comparison between dobutamine and levosimendan for management of post resuscitation myocardial dysfunction. *Critical Care Medicine*, **33**, 487–491.

Kern, K., Hilwig, R., Rhee, K. & Berg, R. (1996) Myocardial dysfunction after resuscitation from cardiac arrest: an example of global myocardial stunning. *Journal of the American College of Cardiology*, **28**, 232–240.

Lucking, S.E., Pollack, M.M. & Fields, A.I. (1986) Shock following generalised hypoxic-ischaemic injury in previously healthy infants and children. *Journal of Pediatrics*, **108**, 359–364.

Mayr, V., Luckner, G., Jochberger, S., *et al.* (2007) Arginine vasopressin in advanced cardiovascular failure during the post-resuscitation phase after cardiac arrest. *Resuscitation*, **72**, 35–44.

Meyer, J., Kern, B., Berg, R.A., *et al.* (2002) Post-resuscitation right ventricular dysfunction: delineation and treatment with dobutamine. *Resuscitation*, **55**, 187–191.

Nolan, J.P., Neumar, R.W., Adrie, C., *et al.* (2008) Post-cardiac arrest syndrome: epidemiology, pathophysiology, treatment, and prognostication. A Scientific Statement from the International Liaison Committee on Resuscitation; the American Heart Association Emergency Cardiovascular Care Committee; the Council on Cardiovascular Surgery and Anesthesia; the Council on Cardiopulmonary, Perioperative, and Critical Care; the Council on Clinical Cardiology; the Council on Stroke. *Resuscitation*, **79**, 350–379.

Paediatric Intensive Care Society (2001) *Standards Document 2001*. Paediatric Intensive Care Society, London.

Resuscitation Council (UK) (2011) *Paediatric Immediate Life Support*, 2nd edn. Resuscitation Council (UK), London.

Studer, W., Wu, X., Siegemund, M., *et al.* (2005) Influence of dobutamine on the variables of systemic haemodynamics, metabolism, and intestinal perfusion after cardiopulmonary resuscitation in the rat. *Resuscitation*, **64**, 227–232.

Takasu, A., Saitoh, D., Kaneko, N., *et al.* (2001) Hyperthermia: is it an ominous sign after cardiac arrest? *Resuscitation*, **49**, 273–277.

Takino, M. & Okada, Y. (1991) Hyperthermia following cardiopulmonary resuscitation. *Intensive Care Medicine*, **17**, 419–420.

Teasdale, G. &Jennett, B. (1974) Assessment of coma and impaired consciousness: a practical scale. *Lancet*, **2**, 81–84.

Tobias, J., Lynch, A. & Garrett, .J (1996) Alterations of end-tidal carbon dioxide during the intrahospital transport of children. *Pediatric Emergency Care*, **12**, 249–251.

Treggiari, M., Karir, V., Yanez, N., *et al.* (2008) Intensive insulin therapy and mortality in critically ill patients. *Critical Care*, **12**, R29.

Vasquez, A., Kern, K., Hilwig, R., *et al.* (2004) Optimal dosing of dobutamine for treating post-resuscitation left ventricular dysfunction. *Resuscitation*, **61**, 199–207.

Zeiner, A., Holzer, M., Sterz, F., *et al.* (2001) Hyperthermia after cardiac arrest is associated with an unfavorable neurologic outcome. *Archives of Internal Medicine*, **161**, 2007–2012.

Chapter 12

Bereavement

Kirsti Soanes

Introduction

The sudden death of a child is probably one of the most stressful clinical scenarios faced by healthcare professionals. Death in childhood goes against the natural order of life expectancy, and it is well documented that the long-term effects on parents and wider family members are profound. Dealing with the death of a child is a very emotive situation for staff, which requires sensitivity, professionalism and empathy.

The successful management of such a tragic and distressing situation requires good teamwork, effective communication between all those involved, set protocols to follow and support for staff. It is essential that family-centred care remains the focus and priority of professionals delivering the care, but sometimes this will occur in conjunction with adhering to legal guidelines that can appear to restrict family interaction with the dead child if the cause of death is unknown. This is why it is vital that the staff caring for the child and family are knowledgeable, are up to date with current guidelines and procedures, and can confidently care for grieving families with compassion while maintaining professional standards.

Due to evolving guidelines and legal procedures, there are now more set policies to follow to ensure that the cause of death is investigated thoroughly and in a timely manner. The

Paediatric Advanced Life Support: A Practical Guide for Nurses, Second Edition.
Phil Jevon.

introduction of Local Safeguarding Children Boards and, from those, Child Death Overview Panels (Department for Education, 2010) means that there is now a prescribed chain of evidence collection and communication to all relevant agencies to try to ensure that cases of abuse are not missed, and that cases in which death could have been prevented are examined for necessary action. These actions cover children and young people aged 0–18 years in cases of sudden death.

The aim of this chapter is to understand the general principles of managing bereavement. If a more comprehensive and detailed account is required, this can be found elsewhere (Dent & Stewart, 2004; Sidebotham & Fleming, 2007, Hindmarch, 2009).

Learning objectives

At the end of this chapter, the reader will be able to:

- Describe an ideal layout for the family room
- Discuss the principles of breaking bad news
- Discuss the principles of telephone notification of family members
- Outline the practical arrangements following a death
- Discuss the importance of written guidelines and policies
- Discuss the issues involved with family members witnessing resuscitation

Ideal layout for the family room

The family room should be near to but not immediately in earshot of or visually connected to the resuscitation area. It should ideally be large enough to incorporate comfortable chairs for several people, space for other children and wheelchair access. If possible, the room should have a window to prevent a feeling of claustrophobia. There should also be:

- Hot and cold drinks, a fridge, a kettle and a non-institutional tea/coffee set
- A telephone with dial-in and dial-out facilities
- Books and toys for children
- Access to toilet facilities
- Tissues

Principles of breaking bad news

Allocation of an experienced nurse

It is recommended that an experienced nurse should be allocated to care for family members. This nurse (Hallgrimsdottir, 2000; Rattrie, 2000) should:

- Be familiar with resuscitation procedures and terminology
- Have good communication skills
- Have good counselling skills
- Be able to undertake this role unsupervised

Who should tell the relatives

If the family are not in the resuscitation room when the child dies, or if they arrive after the death, someone will have to break the news to them. This should be done at the earliest opportunity, thus saving them from waiting in vain and hoping for good news. It is essential that the person breaking the bad news is a senior member of staff, knows the child's name, has been present at the resuscitation and is accompanied by the nurse who has been caring for the family.

Preparation

Adequate preparation is essential. All the relevant child's information, including medical and resuscitation details, should be gathered together. Self-preparation, e.g. washing hands and checking clothing for blood, is also important. The names of the closest family members should be sought.

Dent & Stewart (2004) describe the importance of how the initial care at the time of death can have a long-lasting impact on the family, and have produced a helpful acronym for healthcare staff to use as a preparation guide prior to breaking the bad news (Box. 12.1).

What to tell the family

The way in which bad news is broken is critical. Words such as 'dead' or 'died' are unequivocal and will not be misinterpreted.

Box 12.1 Preparation guide to breaking bad news: the *COMPASSION* approach

Care and compassion are key elements. Do you have these qualities?
Offer yourself as a fellow human being, listening carefully and actively. Remember your body language will convey what you are thinking.
Message of grief: recognise that the pain of grief cannot be taken away. There are no instant solutions and, therefore, no hard and fast rules for how to respond
Preparation is important. Are you ready to care for bereaved families? Do you know where to find information, equipment and who to contact to offer support?
Accept the parent(s) reactions. Can you deal with anger or silence?
Seek help if you feel overwhelmed or out of your depth. Who can you talk to?
Supervision or workplace support should be available to you. Ensure you have time to debrief and learn from each situation.
Information is important to parents and family members. Do you know where to find written information for families?
Offer choices to parent(s) to help make them make informed decisions.
Notify other health professionals and agencies, particularly in primary health, so they can continue the care you have started

Honest direct information about the sequence of events, from practitioners who do not skirt around the real issues, is valued by relatives and prevents confusion (Hindmarch, 2009). If the family do not speak English well enough to hold a conversation, all efforts should be made to find a suitable translator in a timely manner so that information can be exchanged between the family and the healthcare professionals. Although it is not ideal, the use of a telephone translation service could be utilised rather than keeping the family waiting for news.

The family should be told in plain language that the child has died despite all efforts to save his or her life. Phrases such as 'We've lost him', 'She slipped away' or even 'She passed on' can be misleading or misinterpreted, leading to even more distress when the truth is finally realised.

Good communication techniques

Good communication techniques include:

- Introducing yourself and colleague(s)
- Confirming that they are the correct family members and identifying who are the closest members (usually the parents)

- Sitting down in order to be at the same level as the relatives
- Establishing and maintaining eye contact
- Allowing time, not rushing and allowing periods of silence so that the information can be absorbed
- Avoiding platitudes such as 'I know what you are going through'; instead, reflect back on their emotions, e.g. 'It must be a terrible shock for you'
- Answering questions in a sympathetic and non-judgemental way
- Sharing a cup of tea (if appropriate); this can help the relationship (Wright, 1996)

The family members may reach for physical contact, such as holding hands or wanting an arm around their shoulders, or they may withdraw, even avoiding eye contact. It can also be a very emotional time for the staff involved, and family members are often grateful to see this (Hindmarch, 2009). This can convey the message that their child was really cared for by them. Although some display of emotion should not be seen as unprofessional or a sign of weakness, it should not become a situation where the relatives are comforting the staff.

Telephone notification of family members

Telephone notification of family members is rare with child death and is never easy. To minimise confusion and misunderstanding, the information should be clear and concise. It is suggested to:

- Identify yourself and the hospital
- Establish whom you are speaking to – if this is not the key family member, find out where he or she can be found
- Give the name of the child and ward. It seems to be common practice not to inform relatives over the telephone that the child has died, but instead to tell them that the child's condition has deteriorated rapidly, is critical or words to that effect. A dilemma arises if the nurse is asked if the child has died. The author's view is that an honest approach is preferable. Wright (1996) suggests that if the hospital is easily accessible, the relatives should be told when they arrive and not over the phone

- Check that the family are clear about the message and are familiar with how to get to the hospital
- Document the exact details of the telephone conversation

Practical arrangements following a death

Cultural and religious requirements

As part of the family care and the last offices for the child, any specific religious or cultural requirements should be ascertained. It may be necessary to request a hospital chaplain or a local religious leader to be present with the family and child. When a baby has died, the family may wish for him or her to be baptised, and this should be arranged as quickly as possible (Huband & Trigg, 2000). It is useful to keep a list of contacts for the main religions in case the family are unable to provide specific details.

Expressions of grief and handling the body can vary depending on the patient's religion and cultural background. There may also be restrictions on what can be done due to a potential post mortem examination, and this needs to be clarified prior to family involvement in the last offices. The Nursing Times 'Death with Dignity' booklets, which detail specific beliefs and procedures in the event of death for most religions, are very useful. It must be considered however, that all families are individuals despite their cultural or religious beliefs, and it is essential that any cultural or religious observances are discussed with the family, rather than assumptions being made that could potentially cause more distress.

Viewing the child's body

While the family are being informed about the death of their child, the child can be prepared for viewing by nursing staff. In most cases, even for coroner's referrals, medical equipment such as tracheal tubes, intravenous cannulae, intraosseous needles can be removed, but this should be ascertained before it is done. The child should have any obvious blood or other bodily fluids cleaned away, but a thorough wash is not usually necessary and could potentially remove evidence for the coroner. Any wounds should be covered with a dry dressing.

The child should be dressed in their own clothes if suitable; if not, an appropriately sized gown or spare clothes should be used – a shroud is never appropriate. Staff should ensure that the child is laid on and covered by clean sheets, and the room should be private, without risk of intrusion. The child should be positioned supine, and the eyes should be closed. A baby could be laid in a Moses basket to look less clinical.

The family members should be informed of how their child appears before they enter the room, especially if there are obvious injuries. Once in the room, they should be encouraged to hold their child (if they are able) and talk to them if they want to. This allows the grieving process to begin by accepting that their child is dead.

Although the family must never be rushed through this, there has to come a time when they have to leave their child. There should be a protocol regarding how they can return to view their child, perhaps with other family members. When the death is sudden and unexplained, a member of staff must be present with the family at all times. This is an essential part of the legal process and prevents any accusation of evidence-tampering.

Role of the police and coroner

The family should be made aware that the police and the coroner will be informed, and that this is standard practice for all sudden unexplained paediatric deaths. If the child arrived via an emergency ambulance, it is likely that the police will have already been notified. If not, the senior doctor on duty is legally obliged to call them. Most often, the police will return to the address where the child was when he or she collapsed, to collect evidence. This can obviously be very distressing for the family. It is very important to emphasise that this is routine, and that the parents are not necessarily under any suspicion of wrongdoing.

As with all sudden deaths, the doctor in charge of the child's care or the police will refer to the coroner to decide whether a post mortem examination is required. If the coroner decides that a post mortem is required, the family cannot refuse as this is a legal decision. But the family should be reassured over what the examination will entail, and that it will resolve the question of why their child has died. It is very important for the relatives to be told that great care is taken to retain the child's normal appearance, and that the family will be able to view the child again once the post mortem has been performed.

The Foundation for the Study of Infant Deaths has published a very useful leaflet for parents and carers that explains, in layman's terms, the process of investigating a sudden death in childhood. This is available at http://fsid.org.uk/document.doc?id=146 (Foundation for the Study of Infant Deaths, 2010), and it is advisable to keep hard copies of it to give to bereaved families prior to their leaving the department.

As part of the coroner's investigation, it will probably be necessary for the child to have certain investigations performed in the first few hours after death. These can include blood tests, a urine collection, a skin biopsy and skeletal survey X-rays. This is mainly to investigate natural causes of death, such as metabolic disease or genetic disorders, but it can also assist in determining any unnatural cause of death. It is essential that staff keep the clothes that the child was wearing, including the nappy if relevant. The police may take these items as evidence. If not, they should accompany the child to the mortuary, properly labelled.

Documentation

The importance of contemporaneous documentation during a paediatric resuscitation and subsequent death cannot be overemphasised. The allocation of a member of staff to be the nominated 'scribe' allows all pertinent information to be documented as the resuscitation attempt is in process. This then negates the situation of team members trying to document retrospectively, which could lead to errors. In addition, if this information is subsequently required by the coroner or police, it is more likely to be accurate.

It is also an essential requirement that somebody has documented all the pre-hospital information from family members, paramedics or other pertinent sources while it is still a fresh memory. Once death is pronounced, the parents and family members may well be too overwhelmed to give an accurate history of preceding events.

Information for the family

It is essential that family members are given written information regarding the arrangements for their child. At such a distressing time, the family will not be able to remember verbal information, and this could cause them unnecessary confusion and added stress.

The information should include the name and telephone number of a nominated person, such as a bereavement counsellor, or a nominated nurse who can act as a central contact in the event of any queries. In addition, the contact number for the coroner's office, or the police officer assigned to the family, should be given. This advice should also contain information on whom to contact should relatives wish to return to view the child.

It can also be useful to provide the name and telephone numbers of any agencies that can provide support, such as the Foundation for the Study of Infant Death, Child Bereavement Trust or Child Death Helpline.

Before the family leave, it is vital that a thorough medical history of the events that led up to the child's death is taken. This could have been done while the family were waiting during the resuscitation, or it could be done afterwards. It is unlikely that parents will be able to remember specific details at a later time, and accurate record-keeping is essential, especially if there might be an inquest or criminal investigation (Advanced Life Support Group, 2011). It is recommended that families are offered an appointment to return to the hospital to see the responsible medical consultant and/or bereavement team so that they can have medical issues explained, and this also gives the family chance to ask questions or give feedback (Royal College of Paediatrics and Child Health, 2007).

Keep-sakes

Many areas offer the relatives a memorial booklet containing such items as a lock of hair, a photograph and hand- or footprints. It has been shown that such mementoes are well received by the family, but it should be at the discretion of the nurse caring for the family whether they are offered immediately or given at a later time. It should be remembered that if a Polaroid camera is used for photographs, these can fade over time, and this should be mentioned to the family.

Transport arrangements

The nurse caring for the family needs to make travel arrangements to take the relatives home – they should never be allowed to drive themselves.

Communication with other agencies

Communication with other relevant agencies, e.g. the general practitioner or health visitor, and the child's school is essential. These agencies need to be informed about the child's death as soon as possible as they may be able to provide support to family members.

Staff support

Dealing with the sudden death of a child is a very stressful event for all healthcare professionals. There may be a feeling that the team has 'failed' in its resuscitation attempts, or that perhaps they should have tried for longer. Being involved in the attempt to save a child's life is a very emotional and distressing time, and for that reason such resuscitations may be longer due to staff being unwilling to give up.

Due to the nature of the situation, it is vital that staff involved are offered the chance for debriefing. This should be a formal process, facilitated by someone who has the appropriate training and skills required. Ideally, it should include all members of the multidisciplinary team who were involved, and some centres also invite pre-hospital personnel, such as paramedics. This can be the ideal time to raise questions about treatment or procedures, and to receive reassurance about the outcome.

In rare cases, staff will deal with the death of a child where abuse or an unnatural cause is suspected. If this occurs, it is likely that members of the healthcare team involved will be asked for police statements and will then potentially be requested to attend a coroner's court and/or Crown court if a prosecution goes ahead. In this circumstance, the staff involved must be offered formal support by their employing organisation, as the circumstances of the death and the following legal procedures will cause stress and anxiety.

Importance of written guidelines and policies

The key to coping with such situations is to ensure that there are written guidelines and policies to follow. This should facilitate an organised plan of care for both the child and the family, and therefore minimise the distress for both the relatives and the staff. Even if paediatric death is a very rare occurrence, having such written information will be invaluable when dealing with an already fraught event.

Such guidelines and policies should be easily accessible, and all staff should be encouraged to read them regularly, therefore keeping themselves up to date. It is easiest if guidelines take the form of a flowchart as they will then be organised and logical. All local protocols regarding coroner referrals, contact telephone numbers, mortuary arrangements, etc., should be stored with the hospital policies, therefore keeping all the necessary information and relevant paperwork together.

It can be helpful to have nominated staff members who are responsible for the updating this information, and who could also be contact points for other agencies (police, coroner, etc.) when new policies or practices are being introduced.

The Foundation for the Study of Infant Deaths (2005) has provided a useful checklist for A&E staff.

Family members witnessing resuscitation

Benefits

Over the last 10 years or so, family-witnessed resuscitation of children has become common practice in the UK, and increasingly worldwide. There is now a body of evidence to support the advantages of this approach. Family-witnessed resuscitation is helpful (Resuscitation Council (UK), 2010) because it:

- Reinforces the fact that the child has died, avoiding prolonged denial and assisting with the bereavement process.
- Avoids distress that may have been brought on by being separated from the child
- Allows family members to be a part of the decision to stop resuscitation attempts
- Enables the family members to talk to the child
- Allows the family members to see for themselves that everything possible has been done
- Allows the family members to touch and speak with the deceased while the body is still warm

Disadvantages

Disadvantages of family members witnessing resuscitation include that it:

- Could cause distress, particularly if invasive procedures are undertaken
- Might hinder the cardiac arrest team, either physically or emotionally

However, in a review of 32 articles published about the presence of the family during resuscitation, Hodge & Marshall (2009) found little evidence to support the fear of staff that families would hinder the resuscitation.

Necessary safeguards when family members witness resuscitation

If family members witness the resuscitation, it is vital that the allocated family nurse stays with them constantly, explaining procedures, answering questions and observing for signs of their becoming overwhelmed by the situation (Royal College of Paediatrics and Child Health, 2007; Hodge & Marshall, 2009). It should be emphasised that they can leave the room at any time, and that they will be asked to leave if they are becoming too distressed or interfere with the resuscitation attempt.

Summary

Dealing with the sudden death of a child can be deeply stressful for both staff and family members. Healthcare professionals need to know how to support bereaved family members through the process of grieving following a child's death. This chapter has discussed the principles of the early management of bereavement, including how to break bad news. Allowing family members to witness resuscitation can help with the bereavement process.

References

Advanced Life Support Group (2011) *Advanced Paediatric Life Support*, 4th edn. Wiley Blackwell, Oxford.

Dent, A. & Stewart, A. (2004) *Sudden Death in Childhood: Support for the Bereaved Family*. Butterworth Heinemann, Edinburgh.

Department for Education (2010) Working Together to Safeguard Children: A Guide to Inter-agency Working to Safeguard and Promote the Welfare of Children. Retrieved from https://www.education.gov.uk/publications/eOrderingDownload/00305-2010DOM-EN.pdf (accessed November 2011).

Foundation for the Study of Infant Deaths (2005) Suggested Guidelines for Accident and Emergency Departments. Retrieved from http://fsid.org.uk/document.doc?id=9 (accessed November 2011).

Foundation for the Study of Infant Deaths (2010) The Child Death Review: A Guide for Parents and Carers. Retrieved from http://fsid.org.uk/document.doc?id=146 (accessed November 2011).

Hallgrimsdottir, E. (2000) Accident and emergency nurses' perceptions and experiences of caring for families. *Journal of Clinical Nursing*, **9**, 611–619.

Hindmarch, C. (2009) *On the Death of a Child*, 3rd edn. Radcliffe Publishing, Oxford.

Hodge, A. & Marshall, A. (2009) Family presence during resuscitation and invasive procedures. *Collegian*, **16**, 101–118.

Huband, S. & Trigg, E. (2000) *Practices in Children's Nursing: Guidelines for Community and Hospital*. Churchill Livingstone, London.

Rattrie, E. (2000) Witnessed resuscitation: good practice or not? *Nursing Standard*, **14**, 32–35.

Resuscitation Council (UK) (2010) 2010 Resuscitation Guidelines. Retrieved from http://www.resus.org.uk/pages/GL2010.pdf (accessed 20 May 2011).

Royal College of Paediatrics and Child Health (2007) *Services for Children in Emergency Departments*. RCPCH, London.

Sidebotham, P. & Fleming, P. (2007) *Unexpected Death in Childhood: A Handbook for Practitioners*. Wiley & Sons, Chichester.

Wright, B. (1996) *Sudden Death: A Research Base for Practice*, 2nd edn. Churchill Livingstone, New York.

Chapter 13

Records, Record-keeping and Audit

Introduction

An accurate written record detailing the paediatric resuscitation event is essential. It forms an integral part of the medical and nursing management of the child, and can help to protect the practitioner if defence of his or her actions is required.

Unfortunately, the exact timing and sequence of events and interventions can sometimes be difficult to recall. Nevertheless, despite this, accurate record-keeping will still be expected. In addition, an audit of in-hospital resuscitation attempts should be ongoing following national and international guidelines.

The aim of this chapter is to understand the principles of good record-keeping and audit.

Learning objectives

At the end of this chapter, the reader will be able to:

- Discuss the importance of accurate record-keeping
- Outline the principles of effective record-keeping
- Detail what post-resuscitation records should include
- Discuss the uniform reporting of data related to in-hospital resuscitation
- Discuss when records become a legal document
- Outline the National Cardiac Arrest Audit (NCAA)

Paediatric Advanced Life Support: A Practical Guide for Nurses, Second Edition.
Phil Jevon.
© 2012 Phil Jevon. Published 2012 by Blackwell Publishing Ltd.

Importance of accurate record-keeping

Accurate record-keeping will help to protect the welfare of the child by promoting high standards of clinical care and continuity of care through better communication and dissemination of information between members of the interprofessional healthcare team. Accurate records will also help the practitioner to promptly detect any changes in the child's condition.

Principles of effective record-keeping

According to the Nursing and Medical Council (2009), there are a number of factors that contribute to effective record-keeping. Records should:

- Be factual, consistent and accurate
- Be documented as soon as possible after the event
- Provide current information on the care and condition of the patient
- Be documented clearly and in such a way that the text cannot be erased
- Have any alterations and additions dated, timed and signed, with all original entries clearly legible
- Be accurately dated, timed and signed (including a printed signature)
- Not include abbreviations, jargon, meaningless phrases or irrelevant speculation

What post-resuscitation records should include

It is most important that the resuscitation attempt is fully documented in the notes. The following should be included:

- Time of arrest, including presenting ECG rhythm
- Events leading up to the arrest
- Details of resuscitation, including ECG rhythms and response to treatment
- Tracheal intubation time and duration of ventilation

- Details of drugs administered, including the doses and routes used
- Details of defibrillation, particularly the time interval from the recognition of a shockable rhythm to the first shock
- Any pertinent blood chemistry, e.g. arterial blood gases, pH and base deficit results
- The names and designations of personnel present
- Reasons for any delay in starting resuscitation
- Details of communication with the parents
- When resuscitation was stopped, either because it was successful or because it was abandoned

Records as a legal document

There is often concern over what constitutes a legal document. Basically, any document requested by the court becomes a legal document, e.g. nursing records, medical records, X-rays, laboratory reports, in fact any document which may be relevant to the case. If any of the documents are missing, the writer of the records may be cross-examined over the circumstances of their disappearance:

> medical records are not proof of the truth of the facts stated in them but the maker of the records may be called to give evidence as to the truth as to what is contained in them. (Dimond, 2011)

National Cardiac Arrest Audit

The National Cardiac Arrest Audit (NCAA) is a joint initiative between the Resuscitation Council (UK) and the Intensive Care National Audit and Research Centre. Open to all acute hospitals in the UK and Ireland, it aims to identify and foster improvements in the prevention, care delivery and outcomes of cardiac arrest (Resuscitation Council (UK), 2011).

It is an ongoing, national, comparative outcome audit that monitors and reports on the incidence and outcome of in-hospital cardiac arrests in order to inform resuscitation practice and resuscitation policy. The initial scope of data collection is: 'all individuals (excluding neonates) receiving chest compressions and/or defibrillation from the hospital based resuscitation team (or equivalent)', i.e. the team that responds to internal crash call telephone calls (2222) at the hospital (Resuscitation Council (UK), 2011).

Resuscitation data are collected according to standardised definitions and entered onto the NCAA secure web-based system. Once the data have been validated, hospitals are provided with activity reports and comparative reports that will be available online when accessed using a password (Resuscitation Council (UK), 2011).

For further information regarding the NCAA, visit www. icnarc.org or contact the NCAA team by email ncaa@icnarc.org or by telephone: 020 7554 9779.

Summary

This chapter has discussed the importance of accurate record-keeping and outlined the principles underlying effective record-keeping, detailing what post-resuscitation records should include. It has discussed the uniform reporting of data related to in-hospital resuscitation and the point at which records become a legal document. Finally, it described the NCAA.

References

Dimond, B. (2011) *Legal Aspects of Nursing*, 6th edn. Pearson Education, London.
Nursing and Midwifery Council (2009) *Record Keeping: Guidance for Nurses and Midwives*. NMC, London.
Resuscitation Council (UK) (2011) National Cardiac Arrest Audit (NCAA) Overview and Status. Retrieved via www.resus.org.uk (accessed 3 June 2011).

Chapter 14

Legal and Ethical Issues

Richard Griffith

Introduction

Law and ethics are now fundamental to the practice of nursing, including resuscitation. The law informs nursing at every stage, and it is essential that readers understand and are able to critically reflect on the legal issues relevant to practice. This is particularly true in emergency situations when an appropriate and timely response is required.

In treating patients, you undertake a duty of care towards those patients not to harm them, in accordance with the law of negligence. Your right to touch a patient will be based on the law of consent, and the informed and freely given permission of the patient will be a prerequisite to any lawful treatment. The legal principles of confidentiality and negligence regulate the relationship between you and your patients while they are in your care.

The standards of the profession and its regulatory body, the Nursing and Midwifery Council (NMC), are derived from fundamental human rights principles. These principles largely underpin the law relating to healthcare and the standards of conduct and performance required of practitioners by the NMC document *The Code* (Nursing and Midwifery Council, 2008).

The aim of this chapter is to provide an introduction to law and ethics relating to resuscitation.

Paediatric Advanced Life Support: A Practical Guide for Nurses, Second Edition. Phil Jevon.
© 2012 Phil Jevon. Published 2012 by Blackwell Publishing Ltd.

Learning objectives

At the end of this chapter, the reader will be able to:

- Discuss the scope of a nurse's accountability
- Discuss the issues related to Do Not Attempt Resuscitation orders
- List the factors influencing the decision to stop cardiopulmonary resuscitation (CPR)
- Discuss a risk management strategy for CPR

The scope of a nurse's accountability

As a registered nurse, you will be legally and professionally accountable for your actions, irrespective of whether you are following the instructions of another or using your own initiative. Healthcare litigation is increasing, and patients are increasingly prepared to assert their legal rights. It is perhaps little wonder therefore that the NMC insists you are able to practise in accordance with an ethical and legal framework that ensures the primacy of patients' and clients' interests (Nursing and Midwifery Council, 2008).

A thorough and critical appreciation of the legal and professional issues affecting nursing practice is essential if you are to develop the professional awareness necessary to satisfy the NMC that you are an accountable practitioner, competent to practise as a registered nurse. The advantages of legal awareness are listed in Box 14.1.

Defining accountability

In their seminal work on the subject, Lewis and Batey (1982) defined accountability as:

> the fulfilment of a formal obligation to disclose to referent others the purposes, principles, procedures, relationships, results, income and expenditures for which one has authority.

An analysis of Lewis and Batey's definition reveals the fundamental nature of accountability. The 'fulfilment of a formal

Box 14.1 The advantages of legal awareness for the nurse professional

The legally aware nurse:

- Realises that many aspects of daily life are governed by law
  Most aspects of life are regulated by law. Legal awareness helps you appreciate the importance of the legal framework that supports the structure of society
     It also allows you to appreciate that personal and social problems may have a legal dimension
- Knowingly acts in accordance with legal principles
  Many parts of the law are necessarily complex and difficult to understand. However, the underlying principles are quite simple. These affect everyone on a day-to-day basis, and therefore an understanding of them is important. Indeed, ignorance of the law can bring very serious consequences.
- Understands the key elements of the legal system
  Knowledge of the law is of limited value unless you understand the various ways in which the legal system works to enforce the law
     It is important to understand the role of those agencies which have powers to enforce the law, and of the mechanisms by which you can seek legal help and advice
- Knows when and where to seek appropriate advice
  The law is vast and constantly changing. You need to develop a sense of:
    - a) when the law can help or hinder
    - b) what you can find out for yourself and where
    - c) when you should seek expert help
    - d) how to get the appropriate help or advice.
- Understands the nature of law
  Even though many day-to-day situations have a legal dimension, there are some problems that the law can do little about, even when in theory this should not be the case

obligation' suggests that accountability has its basis in law. That is, there is a formal or legal relationship between the practitioner and higher authorities (the 'referent others') that are entitled to hold the practitioner to account. The extent of the scrutiny is illustrated by the inclusion of 'the purposes, principles, procedures, relationships, results, income and expenditures for which one has authority' in the definition. Put more concisely, to be accountable is to be answerable for the acts and omissions within one's practice.

This is the approach adopted by the NMC (2008), the profession's regulatory body, which states in *The Code* (p. 2):

> As a professional, you are personally accountable for actions and omissions in your practice and must always be able to justify your decisions.

> **Box 14.2** The functions of accountability
>
> - *Protective function* – the purpose of accountability is to protect the public from the acts or omissions of nurses that might cause harm
> - *Deterrent function* – the threat of sanction available to the higher authorities against registered practitioners is seen as protecting the public by deterring acts or omissions that might cause harm
> - *Regulatory function* – by making practitioners accountable to a range of higher authorities, the law regulates their behaviour and allows action to be taken to protect the public should they breach the regulatory framework
> - *Educative function* – accountability has an educative function in that those found liable have their cases heard in public with a view to reassuring society that only the highest standards of practice will be tolerated. Other practitioners will learn from such cases and refrain from acting in a similar manner

Functions of accountability

Accountability has four functions which are set out in Box 14.2.

Accountable to whom?

Nurses owe a formal obligation to answer for their practice to a range of higher authorities. These have a legal relationship with nurses that enable them to demand that they justify their practice. If they fail to satisfy those requirements, sanctions may be applied against them.

In order to provide maximum protection to the public, four areas of law are drawn together and can individually or collectively hold practitioners to account (Fig. 14.1).

Accountability to society

Nurses are subject to the same laws as any other member of society, and there is nothing about nurses' status that exempts them from these laws. If nurses are suspected of committing a crime during the course of their practice or otherwise, they can be called to account.

Accountability to society is achieved through the public law. Many of these laws are derived from Acts of Parliament such as the Road Traffic Act 1988, the Theft Act 1968 or the Offences Against the Person Act 1861. Such Acts are known as public general acts, and it is entirely possible to breach them in the course of a practitioner's practice.

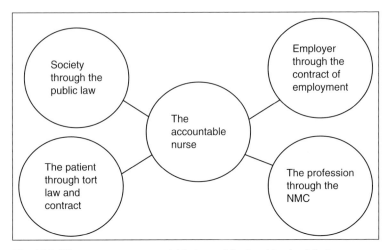

Fig. 14.1 Who nurses are accountable to, and the legal basis of that relationship.

The treatment nurses provide to their patients often requires interventions that are personal and intimate in nature. The public law demands that such interventions are only carried out when it is convincingly shown to be medically necessary and by staff who are properly qualified (*R* v. *Tabassum* [2000]). Where this occurs, the nurse's actions stand outside the criminal law (*Airedale NHS Trust* v. *Bland* [1993]). However, the nurse's acts will lose their immunity if the necessity cannot be made out or the treatment proceeds without either the consent of a capable patient or the best interests of an incapable patient.

The public law seeks to protect patients through the regulation of practice and the environment of care. The National Health Service Litigation Authority (2007) estimates that some £500 million is paid annually by the health service in compensation claims and fines for breaching health and safety laws. The cost in human terms can also be high. Mistakes and errors can compromise safety to the point where lives are put at risk and fatalities do, sadly, occur.

To prevent the avoidable loss of life and minimise the days lost to absence, an employer has a legal duty to comply with the requirements relating to Health and Safety at Work etc Act 1974.

Accountability to the patient

As well as being accountable to society in general, nurses are accountable to the individual patients in their care. The tort or civil law system allows patients to sue for compensation if they believe that harm has been caused through carelessness. Liability for carelessness is given its legal expression in the law relating to negligence.

Negligence is a civil wrong and best defined as actionable harm. That is, a person sues for compensation because he or she has been harmed by the carelessness of another person. Negligence in the healthcare setting has developed under the common law by judges setting rules through decided cases.

In certain circumstances, called duty situations, the nature of the relationship between people gives rise to a duty of care. For example, a manufacturer owes a duty to the consumer of his product (*Donoghue* v. *Stevenson* [1932]), and one road user owes a duty of care to the other road users in his vicinity (*Rouse* v. *Squires* [1973]). Similarly, the nurse–patient relationship gives rise to a duty of care (*Kent* v. *Griffiths* [2001]). Nurses owe their patients a duty of care and are accountable to patients if they cause harm by breaching that duty.

In civil law, nurses are expected to meet the standard of care set by reference to *Bolam* v. *Friern HMC* [1957]. Known as the Bolam test, this requires that nurses meet the standard of the ordinary skilled person exercising and professing to have that special skill or art (*Gold* v. *Haringey HA* [1998]).

Case law demonstrates that the standard covers the whole of the professional relationship with the patient and includes direct care (*Bayliss* v. *Blagg & another* [1954]), advice-giving and record-keeping (*Greenfield* v. *Irwin (A Firm)* [2001]), including even the standard of handwriting (*Prendergast* v. *Sam and Dee* [1989]). If the nurse's actions were in keeping with a respected body of professional opinion, practice will not have fallen below the standard required in law and there will be no liability in negligence (*Bolam* v. *Friern HMC* [1957]). This will be the case even if there were different ways of performing a task under scrutiny. A judge cannot find negligence just because he prefers one professional's view over another's (*Maynard* v. *West Midlands RHA* [1984]).

However, in *Bolitho* v. *City & Hackney HA* [1997], the House of Lords held that any expert evidence used to support a nurse's actions must stand up to logical analysis. That is, the existence of a common practice does not necessarily mean that it is not negligent. A defendant will not be exonerated because others too are negligent or common professional practice is slack.

The duty of care to the patient also requires nurses to keep their knowledge up to date throughout their career (*Roe* v. *Ministry of Health* [1954]). It is most important to attend regular paediatric resuscitation training sessions. The Resuscitation Council (UK) guidelines for resuscitation are revised on a regular basis – it is important to be aware of current resuscitation practice recommendations.

Nurses continue to owe their patients a duty of care in emergency situations such as resuscitation. They are expected to be able to respond effectively to the common emergencies that might arise in their clinical area, and are expected to ensure that their practice is up to date and evidence-based (*Reynolds* v. *North Tyneside Health Authority* [2002]). In relation to treatment decisions taken in an emergency, a nurse will not be found negligent simply because the reasonably competent nurse would have made a different decision, given more time and information.

In *Wilson* v. *Swanson* (1956), the Supreme Court of Canada held that there was no negligence when a surgeon had to make an immediate decision on whether to operate during an emergency, when the operation was subsequently found to have been unnecessary. Moreover, the skill required in the execution of treatment may be somewhat lower because an emergency may overburden the available resources, and if practitioners are forced by circumstances to do too many things at once, the fact that one of them might be done incorrectly would not lightly be taken as negligence.

Although legal proceedings for carelessness are usually instigated in civil law, it is possible to face criminal prosecution where gross negligence has occurred. In *R* v. *Misra & Srivasta* [2004], the Court of Appeal stated that a health professional would be told that grossly negligent treatment that exposed a patient to the risk of death, and caused it, would constitute manslaughter. In this case, two doctors refused to call for timely assistance when informed by nurses that a patient was severely ill. The patient died of toxic shock and the doctors were given 14 month suspended jail terms.

Accountability to the employer

Nurses are accountable to their employer through the contract of employment. The contract sets out the terms and conditions of employment and the standard of work expected of the employee (Rideout, 1983). Many of these terms, for example salary, holiday entitlement, hours of work, etc., are written in the contract and are known as express contract terms.

In addition, many conditions that regulate the relationship between employer and employee are not expressly written into the contract but are there by virtue of decided cases or employment-related legislation. These are known as implied contract terms and include a warranty from the employees to the employer that they will carry out their duties with due care and diligence (*Harmer* v. *Cornelius* (1858)).

Employers are liable for any compensation payable as a result of a civil wrong committed by an employee during the course of their employment as a result of vicarious liability. Employers will wish to minimise that liability, and are entitled under contract law to hold their employees to account through reasonable disciplinary procedures. For nurses, their employer is the most likely authority to hold them to account, as a patient with a grievance is more likely to complain to the employer than take legal action.

In addition, employment law allows a lower burden of proof when deciding whether an employee is guilty of misconduct. Unlike criminal law, where the prosecution must prove a case beyond reasonable doubt or civil law, and where a person must show on the balance of probability that a tort was committed against them, employment law only requires that an employer hold an honest and genuine belief that the employee is guilty of misconduct based on the outcome of a reasonable investigation (*British Home Stores Ltd* v. *Burchell* [1980]).

Accountability to the profession

Nurses are accountable to the profession through the provisions of the Health Act 1999 (Department of Health, 1999). The NMC's role is to protect the public by establishing standards of education, training, conduct and performance for nurses, who must be registered with the Council in order to practise.

The NMC is concerned with protecting the public rather than dealing with local issues such as a breach of employment contract. Only where the conduct or performance of a nurse gives rise to concern for public safety will the NMC become involved. 'Fitness to practise' is the term now used by the NMC to describe a registrant's suitability to be on the register without restrictions. The NMC has the power to hold a registered nurse to account if it is alleged that their fitness to practise is impaired.

The standards by which practitioners are judged and which the NMC considers the public are entitled to expect are set out in *The Code* (Nursing and Midwifery Council, 2008). Practitioners who appear before the NMC's fitness to practise panels are held to account against those standards. The standard of conduct and competence expected by the NMC is that of the average practitioner, not the highest possible level of practice. This approach is similar to that adopted by civil law when judging a skilled practitioner under the Bolam test to determine whether liability in negligence has arisen. The key difference between negligence law and professional accountability, however, is that no action in negligence can occur without harm to the patient. However, a breach of the code can occur and a practitioner can be held to account even though there has been no harm to a patient.

Issues related to Do Not Attempt Resuscitation orders

The main purpose of medical treatment is to benefit the child by restoring or maintaining health as far as possible, thereby maximising benefit and minimising harm. If treatment fails or ceases to be beneficial, it may not be in the best interests of the child to undertake CPR. As the British Medical Association, Resuscitation Council and Royal College of Nursing (2007) state:

> Ideally, clinical decisions relating to children and young people should be taken within a supportive partnership involving patients, their families and the healthcare team. Where CPR may re-start the heart and breathing for a sustained period but there are doubts about whether the potential benefits outweigh the burdens, the views of the child or young person should be taken into consideration in deciding whether it should be attempted.

It is therefore important to identify any child for whom cardiac arrest represents a terminal event in his or her illness and in whom CPR is inappropriate. It is also important to identify any competent child who does not want CPR to be attempted and who competently refuses it.

When discussing a Do Not Attempt Resuscitation (DNAR) order, it is important to consider:

- The likely clinical outcome, including the chances of success-fully restarting the child's heart and breathing, and the overall benefit achieved from successful CPR
- The child's wishes – these are an essential element of the decision
- The child's human rights (see below)
- The parents' wishes

The views of children and young people should be taken into account when considering a DNAR order (British Medical Association *et al.*, 2007). Competent young people can consent to medical treatment, and when they lack competence, it is usually the parents who act on their behalf.

In England, Wales and Northern Ireland, medical staff are not necessarily bound by refusals of treatment by young people because the courts have ruled that consent from people with parental responsibility, or from the court itself, still allows medical staff to provide treatment (British Medical Association *et al.*, 2007). In Scotland, however, it is probable that a competent young person's decision can not be overridden by the courts or by those with parental responsibility (British Medical Association *et al.*, 2007).

If disagreement persists despite attempts to reach an agreement, it is recommended that legal advice is sought (British Medical Association *et al.*, 2007). It must be stressed that medical staff do not have to bow to demands from parents to provide treatment contrary to their professional judgement, although they will often try to accommodate parents' wishes as far as possible as long as the parents are still acting in the best interests of the child (British Medical Association *et al.*, 2007).

The Human Rights Act 1998 and DNAR orders

The Human Rights Act 1998 incorporates the majority of the rights set out in the European Convention on Human Rights into

UK law. In order to meet their obligations under the Act, health professionals must be able to demonstrate that their decisions are compatible with the human rights identified in the Articles of the Convention. Provisions particularly relevant to DNAR orders include the right to:

- Life (Article 2)
- Be free from inhuman or degrading treatment (Article 3)
- Respect for privacy and family life (Article 8)
- Freedom of expression (Article 10)
- Be free from discriminatory practices in respect of these rights (Article 14)

Who makes the decision?

It is widely recognised that any medical decisions relating to children and young people should ideally be taken within a supportive partnership involving them, their families and the healthcare team (British Medical Association *et al.*, 2007). The clinician in charge of the child's care is ultimately responsible for making a DNAR decision (British Medical Association *et al.*, 2007). The views of other members of the healthcare team, the child and the child's parents should also be sought.

Documentation

Once a DNAR order has been made, 'Not for attempted cardiopulmonary resuscitation' should be documented in the medical notes (British Medical Association *et al.*, 2007). The entry should be signed and dated, and should include the rationale behind the order, who was consulted and when it should be reviewed.

The DNAR order should also be documented in the nursing notes by the primary nurse or most senior member of the nursing team, whose responsibility it is to communicate the decision to other members of the nursing team. Accurate record-keeping is essential; it will help to protect the welfare of the child by promoting better communication and dissemination of information between members of the interprofessional healthcare team. The British Medical Association, Resuscitation Council (UK) and Royal College of Nursing have published a helpful flow chart to guide practitioners through the decision-making process.

Factors influencing the decision to stop CPR

Resuscitation is unlikely to be successful if there has been no return of spontaneous circulation despite 20 minutes of quality CPR. Prolonged CPR should be carried out if there is a history of poisoning, hypothermia or persistent ventricular fibrillation/ pulseless ventricular tachycardia (Resuscitation Council (UK), 2011).

Risk management strategy for CPR

> Professionals can take a risk management approach to litigation which on the one hand ensures high standards of care and on the other high standards of evidence should litigation be threatened. (Henderson & Jones, 1996).

Henderson & Jones (1996) have described the key components of a risk management strategy to minimise the risk of litigation:

- Standards of care
- Using protocols
- Monitoring practice
- Identifying risk activities
- Keeping records
- Responding to complaints
- Maintaining a safe environment

Each will now be discussed in turn in the context of paediatric resuscitation.

Standard of care

The law and the public will expect the practitioner to have attained a recognised standard of care that would be expected from any competent healthcare professional. The practitioner will therefore need to keep up to date with current guidelines and strive to ensure that practice is whenever possible based on evidence. This will, of course, require not only knowledge, but also, and certainly more importantly, competency in resuscitation skills. This is where in particular training and regular updates in

CPR techniques are essential if this required level of competency is to be not only reached, but also maintained. Current Resuscitation Council (UK) guidelines for paediatric resuscitation should be followed.

There should also be an audit system in place to ensure that these standards are being achieved and maintained. One objective method of undertaking this is through scenario-testing using a manikin, preferably in the clinical area, following Resuscitation Council (UK) guidelines. It is more beneficial if the team approach to CPR is evaluated, and it is therefore desirable to encourage participation of the crash team members. This will help ensure a more realistic CPR situation.

Protocols

Protocols, e.g. who should attend a CPR attempt, can help to reduce the risk of error and help to ensure that the desired standard of care is delivered. Where appropriate, protocols should be based on current research, guidelines and recommendations, and should be determined and agreed locally. It is important to ensure that all practitioners who will be expected to adhere to them are involved in their production. This will help to ensure that they are followed.

Monitoring practice

All CPR attempts should be audited (see Chapter 13). This can be done by either completing a standard audit form immediately following the event (which is preferable) or by retrospectively by reviewing the child's notes. The main purpose of the audit is to identify any problems, e.g. with equipment or with the resuscitation procedure, and rectify them accordingly. In addition, potential problems may also be highlighted.

Identifying risk activities

Risk activities should be identified; for example, the decision of when to request senior medical support during CPR is one area of clinical practice that is prone to or favours successful litigation. It is important to ensure that regular training is undertaken and appropriate protocols are in place and regularly reviewed.

Keeping-records

Keeping clear comprehensive records is part of the duty of care owed to the patient (Nursing and Midwifery Council, 2008). In addition, records are invaluable when providing evidence in cases of litigation. It is therefore imperative to ensure that high standards of record-keeping are maintained.

Responding to complaints

Complaints should ideally be investigated and settled at an early stage, hopefully preventing them from turning into formal complaints. In addition, good communication and explanations may reduce the incidence of complaints in the first place.

Maintaining a safe environment

The requirements of the Health and Safety at Work etc Act 1974 should be followed. Particular care should be taken with sharps and body fluids. Regular checks should be carried out on the CPR equipment following the manufacturers' recommendations, and any faults or defects should be reported and rectified.

Summary

This chapter has provided an introduction to law and ethics relating to paediatric resuscitation. The scope of the nurse's accountability has been discussed. The issues related to DNAR orders have been outlined, and the factors influencing the decision to stop CPR have been listed. A suggested risk management strategy for CPR has been outlined.

References

Airedale NHS Trust v. *Bland* [1993] AC 789.
Bayliss v *Bragg & another* (1954) 1 BMJ 709.
Bolam v. *Friern HMC* [1957] 1 WLR 582.
Bolitho v. *City & Hackney HA* [1997] 3 WLR 1151.
British Home Stores Ltd v *Burchell* (1980) ICR 303 (EAT).

British Medical Association, Resuscitation Council (UK) & RCN (2007) *Decisions Relating to Cardiopulmonary Resuscitation. A Joint Statement from the British Medical Association, the Resuscitation Council (UK) and the Royal College of Nursing.* BMA, London.

Department of Health (1999) *Health Act 1999.* HMSO, London.

Donoghue v. Stevenson [1932] AC 562.

Gold v. *Haringey HA* [1998] QB 481.

Greenfield v *Irwin (A Firm)* (2001) EWCA Civ 113.

Harmer v. *Cornelius* (1858) 5 CB 236.

Henderson, C. & Jones, K. (1996) *Essential Midwifery*, Mosby, London.

Kent v. *Griffiths* [2001] QB 36 ((CA)).

Lewis, F.M. & Batey, M.V. (1982) Clarifying autonomy and accountability in nursing services. *Journal of Nursing Administration*, **12**(9), 13–18.

Maynard v *West Midlands RHA* [1984] 1 WLR 634 ((HL)).

National Health Service Litigation Authority (2007) *Annual Report and Accounts 2007.* NHSLA, London.

Nursing and Midwifery Council (2008) *The Code: Standards of Conduct, Performance and Ethics for Nurses and Midwives.* NMC, London.

Prendergast v. *Sam and Dee* (1989) 1 Med LR36.

R v. *Misra & Srivasta* [2004] EWCA Crim 2375.

R v. *Tabassum* [2000] 2 Cr App R 328.

Reynolds v. *North Tyneside Health Authority* [2002] Lloyd's Rep Med 459.

Rideout, R.W. (1983) *Principles of Labour Law.* Sweet & Maxwell, London.

Roe v. *Ministry of Health* [1954] 2 QB 66 ((CA)).

Rouse v. *Squires* [1973] 2 All ER 903.

Wilson v. *Swanson* (1956) 5 DLR (2d) 113 (Canadian Supreme Court).

Chapter 15
Resuscitation Training

I hear and I forget, I see and I remember, I do and I understand. (Chinese Proverb)

Introduction

Factors underpinning survival from cardiac arrest include high-quality scientific evidence informing the resuscitation guidelines, the effectiveness of education, and resources for implementing the guidelines (Chamberlain & Hazinski, 2003), as well as how easily the guidelines can be applied in clinical practice and the effect of human factors on putting the theory into practice (Yeung & Perkins, 2010).

Cardiopulmonary resuscitation (CPR) employs skills that are essentially practical, and practitioners need hands-on practical training both to acquire and to maintain them. The methods used to teach CPR techniques have been the subject of much investigation in recent years. Teachers and educationalists has been devoted considerable effort to determining the optimum method of teaching CPR techniques, so that the necessary skills are both acquired and easily retained.

The aim of resuscitation training is to equip learners with the necessary knowledge and skills to perform CPR at a level at which they would be expected to perform, whether they are lay rescuers, first responders or members of the cardiac arrest team

Paediatric Advanced Life Support: A Practical Guide for Nurses, Second Edition.
Phil Jevon.
© 2012 Phil Jevon. Published 2012 by Blackwell Publishing Ltd.

(Baskett *et al.*, 2005). Paediatric resuscitation training needs to be realistic and life-like, particularly as paediatric cardiac arrests occur so infrequently and opportunities to gain practical experience in paediatric resuscitation are limited.

The aim of this chapter is for readers to understand the principles of resuscitation training.

Learning objectives

At the end of this chapter, the reader will be able to:

- Discuss why resuscitation training is important
- List the recommendations for resuscitation training
- Outline the principles of adult learning
- Describe the methods of resuscitation training
- Provide an overview of nationally recognised courses in paediatric resuscitation
- State the key learning objectives of paediatric resuscitation training
- Describe what training manikins and models are currently available for resuscitation training

Why resuscitation training is important

Competence in resuscitation skills

Healthcare practitioners' skills in resuscitation are often very poor (Wynne *et al.*, 1987; Buss *et al.*, 1993).

Healthcare staff's perception of competency at resuscitation

There is a considerable disparity between perceived competence and the actual ability to undertake effective resuscitation (Smith & Hatchett, 1992). In addition, the experience of senior practitioners attending cardiac arrests is that confidence levels are often high, but that these are generally not matched by high skill levels (Wynne *et al.*, 1987).

Retention of skills

The majority of studies have demonstrated that CPR skills, e.g. calling for help, and chest compressions and ventilations, decay within 3–6 months after the initial training session (Berden *et al.*, 1993; Woollard *et al.*, 2004, 2006; de Vries & Handley, 2007; Spoone *et al.*, 2007; Andresen *et al.*, 2008; Smith *et al.*, 2008).

Recommendations concerning resuscitation training

The International Liaison Committee on Resuscitation (Soar *et al.*, 2010) has made the following recommendations concerning resuscitation training:

- Resuscitation training should be evaluated to ensure that it reliably achieves the learning objectives. The aim is to ensure that learners acquire and retain the skills and knowledge that will enable them to act correctly in actual cardiac arrests and improve patient outcomes.
- Short video/computer self-instruction courses, with minimal or no instructor coaching, combined with hands-on practice, can be considered as an effective alternative to instructor-led basic CPR and automatic external defibrillator (AED) training.
- As resuscitation knowledge and skills deteriorate in as little as 3–6 months, it is prudent to undertake frequent assessments of healthcare staff to identify those who need refresher training to help maintain their knowledge and skills.
- As CPR prompt or feedback devices improve the acquisition and retention of CPR skills, they should be considered for resuscitation training for both lay persons and healthcare staff.
- Resuscitation training should also include leadership, teamwork, task management and structured communication skills as these will help to improve the performance of CPR and patient care.
- To help improve teamwork, team briefings to plan for resuscitation attempts and debriefings based on the team's actual performance during a simulated or an actual resuscitation attempt should be considered

Principles of adult learning

Adults are usually well motivated to learn once they realise that the course content is relevant to them. Adults generally learn best when they are treated as adults and when their skills, experience and prior knowledge are recognised and utilised.

The teacher can facilitate adult learning in several ways, by (Fuszard, 1995):

- Acting as a resource person and helper
- Explaining points that have not been understood
- Demonstrating principles, concepts and skills
- Challenging the learner's values when appropriate
- Adopting the role of task-masker and evaluator
- Encouraging leaner self-evaluation
- Managing groups of learners effectively and facilitating the pursuit of intellectual questions

Considerable research has been undertaken evaluating the principles of teaching basic and advanced CPR skills and the factors affecting their retention. Both course content and time devoted to practice on manikins will influence skill attainment and the subsequent retention of skills.

Constructive feedback during training is important and should identify not only the students' strong points, which will increase their confidence and motivation, but also any weaknesses or deficiencies that need to be addressed and that require more practice. In the event of poor performance, students should not be ridiculed.

Poor learner motivation, a poor student–teacher relationship and physical and environmental factors can all create barriers to adult learning (Rogers, 1983).

Methods of resuscitation training

There are various methods of providing resuscitation training. The methods chosen will depend on a number of factors, including time allocation, number of instructors, number of students, equipment, facilities and learning objectives. A variety of methods are often used in each training session.

Regardless of the method used, it is recommended that the following three-part approach to facilitating the teaching and learning process be adopted (Resuscitation Council (UK), 2001):

- *Set* – ensure that the environment (lighting, heating, seating arrangements, audiovisual aids, training manikins, etc.) is adequate for training, set the mood, enhance the learners' motivation, state the session objectives and clarify the roles of the teacher and learners.
- *Dialogue* (the main teaching part of the session) – ensure that the content is presented in a clear and logical format and at a level that the learners can understand. Answer learners' questions appropriately, and check that learners have understood the content.
- *Closure* – include time for questions and queries from the learners, provide a concise summary and clearly terminate the session.

A number of key teaching methods can be used in paediatric resuscitation training, some of which will now be outlined.

Lectures

Lectures can be used to revise core material, highlight key points and complement practical stations, but should not replace practical teaching on manikins and models. They also provide a valuable opportunity for group discussion. To help maintain interest, the lecturer should remember the following key points: conciseness, simplicity, eye contact, variations in speed and volume, and the use of personal experience and questions (Bullock *et al.*, 2008).

Skill stations

As CPR involves essentially practical skills, it is important to ensure that any training session allocates plenty of time for these skills to be taught and practised. Skill stations provide an opportunity to learn a skill and debate relevant issues. They should be placed into the context of the overall CPR procedure and be undertaken in small groups (ideally four to six people). They should take into account, and build on, students' prior experience and knowledge.

Shared aspects of teaching, learning and prior experience will promote both positive regard and mutual respect. Positive feedback, encouragement and guidance are also particularly important when teaching practical skills.

Bullock *et al.* (2008) suggest a four-stage approach to teaching a practical skill:

1. *The instructor demonstrates the skill at normal speed* – the skill is carried out at normal speed without explanation and commentary, except for what would normally be said in the clinical situation. This allows the student to observe the procedure carefully without distraction.
2. *The instructor demonstrates the skill again, but this time with a commentary* – the skill is demonstrated again, but with an explanation. It will be broken down into small steps and will generally not be at a normal speed.
3. *The student provides the commentary while the instructor demonstrates the skill* – this stage is used because a skill is more likely to be learned if the student can describe it in detail. If the student is hesitant, the instructor can prompt by leading with the actions. Conversely, confident candidates can describe the different stages of the skill before they are demonstrated. Any errors must be corrected immediately.
4. *The student demonstrates the skill, together with giving a commentary* – each student then talks through and demonstrates the skill. The instructor now has an opportunity to observe each student to ensure they have understood, and are competent at, the skill.

Simulated cardiac arrest scenarios

Simulated cardiac arrest scenarios are a further method of teaching CPR skills. They can help to develop teamwork and help place CPR into context.

The scenarios, which should form a major part of any training session, follow on logically from the teaching and practice of individual skills, e.g. bag-valve-mask ventilation, chest compressions and intraosseous infusions. They are a way of putting everything together in a systematic and meaningful way. There are many advantages to this form of training:

- They are ideal for training in the clinical area.
- They can help to effectively evaluate both an individual and a group performance.

- They allow practitioners to practise their skills and to work as a team managing a paediatric 'cardiac arrest'.
- They can help to bridge the theory–practice gap.
- They can increase efficiency and credibility, improve communication and decision-making and reduce anxiety.

Mock cardiac arrest drills

Mock cardiac arrest drills provide the opportunity to test the individual's and system's responses to cardiac arrest and have been shown to:

- Improve the knowledge of the advanced life support provider (Mikrogianakis *et al.*, 2008)
- Improve skill performance (Farah *et al.*, 2007)
- Improve confidence (Cappelle & Paul, 1996)
- Improve familiarity with the environment (Villamaria *et al.*, 2008)
- Identify common system and user errors (Hunt *et al.*, 2006, 2008)

Using CPR prompt/feedback devices

Resuscitation training sessions that use a prompt/feedback device can improve the performance, acquisition and retention of CPR skills (Soar *et al.*, 2010). It would therefore be worth considering incorporating CPR prompt/feedback devices into a resuscitation training session (Yeung *et al.*, 2009).

Examples of how these devices can be helpful include (Soar *et al.*, 2010):

- *Prompting* – a metronome to provide a guide to the compression rate
- *Feedback* – after-event information based on the effect of an action, such as a visual display of compression depth

Simulation in resuscitation training

Simulation training is an essential component part of resuscitation training (Soar *et al.*, 2010), where it can be and is used in a variety of different ways (Perkins, 2007). Most studies have demonstrated that simulation training on manikins improves knowledge and skills performance in CPR (Mayo *et al.*, 2004; Owen *et al.*, 2006; Campbell *et al.*, 2009; Donoghue *et al.*, 2009).

Discussion groups

Discussion groups, when well organised, are an effective teaching method (Resuscitation Council (UK), 2001). Discussion reflects the method by which adults learn best; i.e. it is an active means of acquiring information (Bullock *et al.*, 2008). Active group participation can result in an enjoyable learning experience.

It is important to clearly define the desired outcome of the session, e.g. to reach a decision or consensus of opinion (a convergent or closed discussion) or to facilitate learners to express and discuss their views (a divergent or open discussion) (Resuscitation Council (UK), 2001).

Nationally recognized courses in paediatric resuscitation

European Paediatric Life Support course

The European Paediatric Life Support course is suitable for healthcare staff who are involved in paediatric resuscitation (both in and out of hospital), i.e. doctors, nurses, emergency medical technicians, paramedics, etc., who have a duty to respond to sick newborn babies, infants and children in their practice (Buss *et al.*, 1993; Carapiet *et al.*, 2001). The course aims to provide attendees with the knowledge and skills required to safely and effective manage a critically ill child during the first hour of illness and to prevent a deterioration to cardiac arrest (Soar *et al.*, 2010).

Ethos
The European Paediatric Life Support course is taught by instructors who have been trained in teaching and assessment. The ethos of European Resuscitation Council courses is to create a positive environment that promotes learning (Soar *et al.*, 2010):

- First names are encouraged among both faculty and candidates in order to reduce apprehension.
- Interactions between faculty and candidates are designed to be positive.

- Teaching is conducted by encouragement with constructive feedback and debriefing on the learner's performance.
- A mentor–mentee system is used to enhance feedback and support for the candidate.

Some stress is inevitable (Sandroni *et al.*, 2005), particularly during assessment, but the aim of the instructors is to enable the candidates to do their best.

Pre-course preparation
A course manual and pre-course multiple choice paper are forwarded to the candidates approximately 4 weeks prior to the start of the course. The candidates are expected to have studied the manual (the multiple choice paper encouraging the candidates to do so).

Candidates attending the course are expected to be competent in paediatric basic life support and in treating foreign body airway obstruction; however, refresher teaching in both skills is included on the course (Soar *et al.*, 2010).

Format and content
The course typically runs over 2 days and consists mainly of small group teaching, with just a few formal lectures. The key topics and skills covered include:

- The causes and mechanisms of cardiorespiratory arrest in neonates and children
- The recognition and treatment of the critically ill neonate, infant or child, and managing cardiac arrest
- Airway management, oxygen therapy, bag-mask ventilation and tracheal intubation
- The log roll and cervical collar placement
- Vascular access
- Safe defibrillation, cardioversion and use of an AED

Assessment
The assessment component of the course comprises:

- Basic life support
- A simulation-based scenario incorporating assessment of the sick child
- Multiple choice questions

For further information, contact the Resuscitation Council (UK) on +44 20 7388 4678 or via www.resus.org.uk.

Paediatric Immediate Life Support course

The course aims to provide attendees with the knowledge and skills required to safely and effective manage a critically ill child during the first few minutes of illness, and to prevent deterioration to cardiac arrest while waiting for expert help to arrive (Soar *et al.*, 2010).

It is ideal for training nurses, emergency medical services personnel and doctors (Soar *et al.*, 2010). From the author's experience, the Paediatric Immediate Life Support course is particularly appropriate for junior doctors, physicians assistants and junior nurses working in A&E departments and paediatrics.

Pre-course preparation
A course manual is forwarded to the candidates approximately 2 weeks prior to the start of the course. The candidates are expected to read the manual.

Format and content
The Paediatric Immediate Life Support is a 1 day course comprising one lecture, hands-on skills and simulation teaching. A particular strength of this course is that the teaching can be tailored to meet the education needs of the attendees. The content of this mainly practical course includes:

- The causes and mechanisms of cardiorespiratory arrest in infants and children
- Recognition and treatment of the critically ill infant or child
- The initial management of cardiac arrest
- Basic airway management, oxygen therapy and bag-mask ventilation
- Intraosseous access

For further information, contact the Resuscitation Council (UK) on +44 20 7388 4678 or www.resus.org.uk.

Assessment
There is continuous ongoing assessment of key skills, e.g. basic life support and basic airway management.

Certification
The certificate is valid for 1 year.

Advanced Paediatric Life Support course

The Advanced Paediatric Life Support course is overseen by the Advanced Life Support Group (ALSG) in Manchester. This very intense course, which covers cardiac, serious illness and trauma emergencies, is aimed at senior medical and nursing staff working regularly with sick children.

The course is run over 3 days (one being online) and comprises lectures, workshops, skill sessions, scenarios and assessments. A course manual is forwarded to the participants approximately 4 weeks prior to the start of the course. For further information, contact the ALSG on +44 161 794 1999 or via www.alsg.org.

Paediatric Life Support course

The Paediatric Life Support course is also overseen by the ALSG in Manchester. This 1 day course is aimed at nurses and medical staff who may be the first to respond in a paediatric emergency.

The course comprises lectures, workshops, skill sessions, scenarios and assessments. Course materials are forwarded to the participants before the start of the course. For further information, contact the ALSG on +44 161 877 1999.

Key learning objectives of paediatric resuscitation training

Detailed below is a suggested (albeit not exhaustive) list of key learning objectives that may help in the provision of CPR training. At the end of the session, the learner will be able to:

- Demonstrate the correct procedure for checking emergency equipment
- Demonstrate the correct procedure for assessing a collapsed, apparently lifeless child
- State the correct procedure for summoning senior help
- Demonstrate the correct procedure for opening and maintaining a clear airway, including the use of suction

- Demonstrate the correct procedure for inserting an oropharyngeal airway
- Demonstrate the correct procedure for bag-valve-mask ventilation, and achieve a chest rise on the manikin
- Demonstrate effective chest compressions in both an infant and child on a manikin, achieving a rate of at least 100 per minute (but not >120 per minute)
- List the equipment required for tracheal intubation
- List four complications of tracheal intubation
- Demonstrate how to attach the cardiac monitor and select lead II
- Demonstrate the correct procedure for intraosseus infusion on a manikin
- Specify the indications for administering adrenaline
- Discuss when CPR should be stopped

Paediatric training manikins and models

Recent technological advances have enabled the manufacture of lifelike training manikins and models. These are transforming training because a greater number of clinical skills can now be demonstrated and practised in a controlled 'classroom' environment. A general overview of what is currently available will now be detailed.

Airway management models

A number of adult airway management manikins are available. Most are anatomically correct in size and detail, and benefit from having realistic landmarks including nostrils, tongue, oro- and nasopharynx, larynx, epiglottis, vocal cords, trachea, oesophagus, inflatable lungs and stomach.

Airway management skills that can be demonstrated and practised include the sizing and insertion of the oropharyngeal airway (Guedel airway), suction and tracheal intubation. It is, however, not possible on some of the manikins to realistically perform face mask ventilation as it is not always necessary to maintain an open airway to achieve a chest rise. Laerdal's Resusci Baby is a good manikin on which to practise this skill because a neutral position is required before a chest rise can be achieved.

Basic life support manikins

Laerdal's Resusci Baby (Laerdal, Norway) is claimed by the manufacturer to be 'the most realistic infant CPR manikin available'. Its features include natural airway obstruction in which a head tilt–chin lift is required to open the airway, and in which overextension of the neck will occlude it. An optional skill guide provides objective feedback on ventilation and chest compression techniques, and a brachial pulse simulator is a standard feature.

Resusci Junior (also from Laerdal) corresponds to a 5-year-old child. It benefits from realistic anatomical features and chest landmarks. A bilateral carotid pulse can be simulated. Optional extras include a skill guide providing objective feedback on CPR technique and a choking kit. In addition, a water rescue version is available. The manikin comes with a handy carrying case that opens out into a useful kneeling mat.

Also available are the basic low-cost infant and child manikins Baby Anne and Little Junior (Laerdal), which can be purchased individually or in a cost-saving pack of four. These allow more hands-on practice, which is particularly important when teaching paediatric CPR as many learners find the techniques difficult to master, and having to practise in front of colleagues can exacerbate the difficulty.

Intraosseous manikins

There are several intraosseous infusion manikins currently available that enable this life-saving skill to be demonstrated and practised. With some, it is even possible to inject and aspirate fluid. Adam,Rouilly's (Sittingbourne, Kent, (UK)) infant intraosseous infusion simulator benefits from palpable key landmarks and enables students to practise the procedure with accuracy and realism.

Advanced life support manikins

Multifunctional advanced life support manikins are ideal for training for the team management of a paediatric cardiac arrest. Features generally include ECG monitoring, basic and advanced airway management including tracheal intubation, defibrillation, intraosseous infusion and drug administration, as well as basic life support. Practitioners can undertake tasks concurrently, providing a more realistic and interactive training session.

Manikin update kits

It is possible to update the older Resusci Baby and Resusci Junior models at a fraction of the cost of purchasing new ones. These manikin update kits, available from Laerdal, include the new and more convenient sanitation system – a disposable airway that minimises clean-up after class, and a removable face that can be either changed or disinfected between students. In addition, a new head undoubtedly improves the manikin's appearance.

Which manikin?

A number of factors need to be taken into account when purchasing a manikin, including the number of staff to be trained and to what level, the venue, storage, the budget and power requirements. It is certainly recommended that the manikin should be seen before purchase to ensure that it will meet training requirements – some companies employ representatives to demonstrate their products, while others offer them on a 'sale or return' basis. It is also advisable to seek advice from the local resuscitation training officer.

Maintenance of manikins

It is important to ensure that the manikins are properly maintained following the manufacturer's recommendations, particularly in relation to sanitation and the prevention of cross-infection. In addition, it is advisable to seek advice from an infection control nurse specialist.

Summary

The importance of resuscitation training has been discussed. CPR skills are generally poor, and regular training and retraining are required to ensure that competence and skills are maintained at a satisfactory level. The availability of lifelike manikins and models enables realistic resuscitation training to be provided.

References

Andresen, D., Arntz, H.R., Grafling, W., *et al.* (2008) Public access resuscitation program including defibrillator training for laypersons: a randomized trial to evaluate the impact of training course duration. *Resuscitation*, **76**, 419–424.

Baskett, P., Nolan, J., Handley, A., *et al.* (2005) European Resuscitation Council Guidelines for Resuscitation 2005 Section 9. Principles of training in resuscitation. *Resuscitation*, **67**(Suppl. 1), S181–S189.

Berden, H.J., Willems, F.F., Hendrick, J., *et al.* (1993) How frequently should basic cardiopulmonary resuscitation training be repeated to maintain adequate skills? *BMJ*, **306**, 1576–1577.

Bullock, I., Davis, M., Lockey, A. & Mackway-Jones, K. (2008) *Pocket Guide to Teaching for Medical Instructors*, 2nd edn. Blackwell Publishing, Oxford.

Buss, P., McCabe, M., Evans, R., *et al.* (1993) A survey of basic resuscitation knowledge among resident paediatricians. *Archives of Disease in Childhood*, **68**, 75–78.

Campbell, D., Barozzino, T., Farrugia, M. & Sgro, M. (2009) High-fidelity simulation in neonatal resuscitation. *Paediatric and Child Health*, **14**, 19–23.

Cappelle, C. & Paul, R. (1996) Educating residents: the effects of a mock code program. *Resuscitation*, **31**,107–111.

Carapiet, D., Fraser, J., Wade, A., *et al.* (2001) Changes in paediatric resuscitation knowledge among doctors. *Archives of Disease in Childhood*, **84**, 412–414.

Chamberlain, D. & Hazinski, M. (2003) Education in resuscitation. *Resuscitation*, **59**, 11–43.

de Vries, W. & Handley, A.J. (2007) A web-based micro-simulation program for self learning BLS skills and the use of an AED. Can laypeople train themselves without a manikin? *Resuscitation*, **75**, 491–498.

Donoghue, A., Durbin, D., Nadel, F., *et al.* (2009) Effect of high-fidelity simulation on pediatric advanced life support training in pediatric house staff: a randomized trial. *Pediatric Emergency Care*, **25**, 139–144.

Farah, R., Stiner, E., Zohar, Z., *et al.* (2007) Cardiopulmonary resuscitation surprise drills for assessing, improving and maintaining cardiopulmonary resuscitation skills of hospital personnel. *European Journal of Emergency Medicine*, **14**, 332–336.

Fuszard, B. (1995) *Innovative Teaching Strategies in Nursing*, 2nd edn. Aspen, Gaithersburg, MD.

Hunt, E., Hohenhaus, S., Luo, X. & Frush, K. (2006) Simulation of pediatric trauma stabilization in 35 North Carolina emergency departments: identification of targets for performance improvement. *Pediatrics*, **117**, 641–648.

Hunt, E.A., Walker, A.R., Shaffner, D., *et al.* (2008) Simulation of in-hospital pediatric medical emergencies and cardiopulmonary arrests: highlighting the importance of the first 5 minutes. *Pediatrics*, **121**, e34–e43.

Mayo, P., Hackney, J., Mueck, J., *et al.* (2004) Achieving house staff competence in emergency airway management: results of a teaching program using a computerized patient simulator. *Critical Care Medicine*, **32**, 2422–2427.

Mikrogianakis, A., Osmond, M.H., Nuth, J., *et al.* (2008) Evaluation of a multidisciplinary pediatric mock trauma code educational initiative: a pilot study. *Journal of Trauma*, **64**, 761–767.

Owen, H., Mugford, B., Follows, V. & Plummer, J.L. (2006) Comparison of three simulation-based training methods for management of medical emergencies. *Resuscitation*, **71**, 204–211.

Perkins, G. (2007) Simulation in resuscitation training. *Resuscitation*, **73**, 202–211.

Resuscitation Council (UK) (2001) *Generic Instructor Course Manual.* Resuscitation Council (UK), London.

Rogers, C. (1983) *Freedom to Learn in the 1980s.* Merrill, Columbus, OH.

Sandroni, C., Fenici, P., Cavallaro, F., *et al.* (2005) Haemodynamic effects of mental stress during cardiac arrest simulation testing on advanced life support courses. *Resuscitation*, **66**, 39–44.

Smith, K.K., Gilcreast, D. & Pierce, K. (2008) Evaluation of staff's retention of ACLS and BLS skills. *Resuscitation*, **78**, 59–65.

Smith, S. & Hatchett, R. (1992) Perceived competence in cardiopulmonary resuscitation, knowledge and skills, amongst 50 qualified nurses. *Intensive and Critical Care Nursing*, **8**, 76–81.

Soar, J., Mancini, M., Bhanji, F., *et al.* (2010) International consensus on cardiopulmonary resuscitation and emergency cardiovascular care science with treatment recommendations. Part 12. Education, implementation, and teams. *Resuscitation*, **81**, 1434–1444.

Spoone, B.B., Fallaha, J.F., Kocierz, L., *et al.* (2007) An evaluation of objective feedback in basic life support (BLS) training. *Resuscitation*, **73**, 417–424.

Villamaria, F., Pliego, J., Wehbe-Janek, H., *et al.* (2008) Using simulation to orient code blue teams to a new hospital facility. *Simulation in Healthcare*, **3**, 209–216.

Woollard, M., Whitfeild, R., Smith, A., *et al.* (2004) Skill acquisition and retention in automated external defibrillator (AED) use and CPR by lay responders: a prospective study. *Resuscitation*, **60**, 17–28.

Woollard, M., Whitfield, R., Newcombe, R., *et al.* (2006) Optimal refresher training intervals for AED and CPR skills: a randomized controlled trial. *Resuscitation*, **71**, 237–247.

Wynne, G., Marteau, T., Johnston, M., Whitely, C.A. & Evans, T. (1987) Inability of trained nurses to perform basic life support. *British Medical Journal* (Clinical Research Edition), **294**, 1198–1199.

Yeung, J. & Perkins, G. (2010) Timing of drug administration during CPR and the role of simulation. *Resuscitation*, **81**, 265–266.

Yeung, J., Meeks, R., Edelson, D., *et al.* (2009) The use of CPR feedback/prompt devices during training and CPR performance: a systematic review. *Resuscitation*, **80**, 743–751.

Index

Paediatric Advanced Life Support: A Practical Guide for Nurses, Second Edition.
Phil Jevon.
© 2012 Phil Jevon. Published 2012 by Blackwell Publishing Ltd.